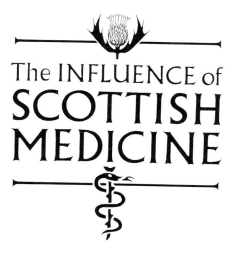

The INFLUENCE of
SCOTTISH
MEDICINE

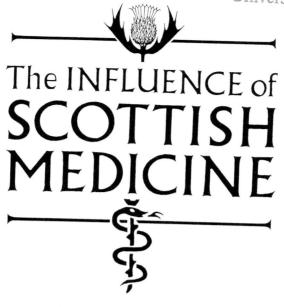

The INFLUENCE of SCOTTISH MEDICINE

*An historical assessment of its
international impact*

Edited by
DEREK A DOW

Published on behalf of the
British Society for the History of Medicine and the
Scottish Society of the History of Medicine

The Parthenon Publishing Group
International Publishers in Science & Technology

Casterton Hall, Carnforth,
Lancs, LA6 2LA, U.K.

120 Mill Road, Park Ridge
New Jersey, U.S.A.

The Proceedings of the 11th British Congress on the History of Medicine, organised by the Scottish Society of the History of Medicine, and held at Edinburgh, 22-24 August, 1986.

The publishers would like to thank Surgikos Limited whose generous financial assistance has made publication of this book possible.

Published in the UK by
The Parthenon Publishing Group Limited
Casterton Hall, Carnforth,
Lancs, LA6 2LA, England

ISBN 1 85070 148 2

Published in the USA by
The Parthenon Publishing Group Inc.
120 Mill Road,
Park Ridge,
New Jersey 07656, USA

ISBN 0 940813 49-1

Printed in Great Britain by
Butler & Tanner Ltd, Frome and London

Contents

The Contributors

Donald Galbraith is a Deputy Keeper in the Scottish Record Office.

John Blair is a Consultant at Perth Royal Infirmary and is currently Vice-President of the Scottish Society of the History of Medicine.

Ronald Girdwood is Professor Emeritus of Therapeutics and Clinical Pharmacology, University of Edinburgh and a Past President of the Royal College of Physicians of Edinburgh.

James Willocks is a Consultant Obstetrician at the Queen Mother's Hospital, Glasgow.

Sir Peter Froggatt was formerly Vice-Chancellor of The Queen's University of Belfast.

Brenda White is a Research Assistant in the Department of Economic History, University of Glasgow.

Andrew Ross is a Senior Lecturer in the History of Missions and former Principal of New College, University of Edinburgh.

David Hamilton is Director of the Wellcome Unit for the History of Medicine, University of Glasgow.

John Aitchison is Professor of Medical Statistics in the University of Hong Kong.

Geoffrey Watson is Professor of Statistics at Princeton University.

Derek Dow is Archivist to the Greater Glasgow Health Board and is currently Joint Honorary Secretary of the Scottish Society of the History of Medicine.

Kenneth Collins is a General Practitioner in Glasgow and a Research Associate of the Wellcome Unit for the History of Medicine.

Thomas Thomson is a Past President of the Royal College of Physicians and Surgeons of Glasgow and is currently Chairman of the Greater Glasgow Health Board.

Introduction

D A Dow

In seeking to draw up a coherent programme for the 11th British
Congress of the History of Medicine, held in Edinburgh from 22-24
August 1986, the SSHM organisers agreed on the theme of 'Medicine
Furth of Scotland' as that most appropriate to the occasion. Scottish
medical schools have for more than two centuries played a role in
global health care out of all proportion to the size of our country or
its population. Despite these achievements there has been no previous
attempt to assess this collective impact. JD Comrie's chapter on 'The
Influence of Scottish Graduates Outside Scotland in the Nineteenth
Century' provided a skeleton which has never been satisfactorily
clothed.[1] This collection of essays will, it is hoped, go some way
towards redressing the balance.

Hume Brown, the doyen of Scottish historians of his time, has
described how the Scot in early times was 'known in Europe as a
student, a scholar, a soldier of fortune, or a trader. *Scotus Viator*, he
was called in Latin — "the wandering Scot."'[2] One of the most
enterprising of these figures was Michael Scot, a mediciner by
profession and reputedly the personal physician to the Emperor
Frederick II. Donald Galbraith provides a lucid and erudite account of
Scot's career, placing the Scottish links with medieval medicine into
a European context.

Writing of the Scot abroad more than a century ago, John Hill
Burton stressed and praised the role of the Scot as a mercenary soldier
through the centuries.[3] John Blair's paper on the Scots and military
medicine reminds us that there was another and more humane side to
the Scottish presence on or near the battlefield. Scottish doctors first
made their mark in naval medicine, and it was superiority on the seas

which created the First British Empire in North America in the 17th
and 18th centuries. Ronald Girdwood's paper traces the influence of
Edinburgh medicine on these new territories in the American and
Canadian colonies.

The impact of Scottish medicine on other nations has not necessarily
involved overseas travel. In his recent volume of *The New History of
Scotland*, Bruce Lenman pays tribute to the influence of three Lanark
men (Smellie, and the Hunter brothers) on London medicine in the mid
18th century. Lenman describes William Hunter as an anatomist, and
makes no reference to the obstetrical achievements of these great
Scottish entrepreneurs.[4] This imbalance is corrected by James
Willocks' contribution on three of the outstanding figures in the
emergence of the 'Man-Midwife' — William Smellie, James Douglas
and William Hunter.

In addition to exporting doctors, the Scottish medical schools in the
18th and 19th centuries attracted large numbers of students. Nowhere
was this trend more marked than in the exodus of Ulster Presbyterians
to study in their spiritual homeland, as clerics or as doctors. In the last
quarter of the 18th and the first quarter of the 19th centuries, both
Scottish and English-born MDs of the Universities of Edinburgh and
Glasgow were outnumbered by those of Irish extraction. Peter
Froggatt's account of the rise and decline of this movement places it
firmly in the context of the creation and expansion of an indigenous
medical school in Belfast.

If the 18th century Scottish doctor had been attendant on the birth
of English obstetrics, his 19th century counterpart had an equally
valuable role to perform in the development of the English public
health movement. Brenda White attributes this evolution to the
peculiarly Scottish amalgamation of public health with 'medical police'
or forensic medicine, a combination which was never adopted south
of the border.

Almost all historians of 19th century Scotland have acknowledged
the contribution of Scotsmen and women to the Christian missionary
outreach, epitomised in David Livingstone's heroic endeavours in
Africa. Few, however, have even mentioned Livingstone's role as a
missionary doctor, concentrating almost entirely on his work as an
explorer.[5] Andrew Ross supplies a timely reminder that a high
proportion of the Scottish missionaries offered cure of the body as well
as the soul, citing the particular contributions of Dr David Livingstone
and Dr Neil MacVicar in South Africa.

The great expansion of Scottish medical influence arguably stemmed from advances in thought during the Scottish Englightenment, a theme which forms the basis of David Hamilton's paper. It was during this same era that the Scots began to play a dominant role in the affairs of the Indian Empire, thanks largely to the influence of Henry Dundas.[6] The Indian Medical Service was a particularly fruitful field for Scottish endeavour. John Aitchison and Geoff Watson have compiled a fascinating and unusual case study of the contribution made to our understanding of the epidemiology of malaria by the mathematical genius of Anderson Gray McKendrick.

Joseph Lister's genius is unquestioned but the true extent of his influence on a generation of Scottish doctors has yet to be analysed. A preliminary assessment of this kind forms one of the themes of Derek Dow's paper on Scotland and Australasia.

Comrie's volume, published in 1932, had little to say about Scotland's 20th century contributions to medicine. Christopher Harvie's volume of *The New History of Scotland* is even more uncommunicative, containing no references to the Scots abroad or to the medical profession *per se*.[7] Despite this desire to keep our light hidden under a bushel, Scottish medical education was highly regarded at the beginning of the 20th century. No less a figure than Abraham Flexner, a respected authority in American medical circles, returned from his European tour in 1912 deeply impressed by the methods and techniques of the Glasgow University medical school.[8] This reputation, and the absence from Scotland of the discriminatory quotas imposed in their homeland, were contributory factors in the incredible influx to Scotland of American Jews in search of a medical education during the inter-war years. Kenneth Collins has done a fine job in resurrecting this largely forgotten episode and recording the impressions of many of the participants.

While history is essentially backward-looking, the role of the Scots in medicine world-wide is by no means over. The final paper in this collection, by Thomas Thomson, describes the current work of the three Royal Medical Colleges in Scotland in the teaching and examination of overseas medical students, especially at the postgraduate level.

This volume is, of course, by no means exhaustive. Entire countries — even continents — have been omitted from our studies. In some cases, notably with regard to Russia, the significant work of the Scots has already been recorded.[9] Little has yet been written about the

Scots in other parts of the globe. In China, as in other parts of the Far East, Scottish missionary doctors played a crucial role in the introduction of Western Medicine. The most important achievement in this field was undoubtedly the establishment by Dugald Christie of the Moukden Medical College.[10] In a similar context, Patrick Manson, an Aberdeen graduate, was instrumental as early as 1887 in founding a medical college for Chinese students in Hong Kong.[11] In Japan, Dr Henry Faulds made important contributions to forensic medicine through his work on fingerprinting techniques,[12] while William Willis, an Irishman educated at Glasgow University, had a large share in the establishment of the first medical school and hospital in the capital of Japan after the restoration of the Meija dynasty.[13]

In another sphere — the West Indies, Central and South America — the contribution of the Scottish doctor appears to be even more neglected by historians. Little is recorded, for example, about the work of James Ramsay who provided medical care to the slave population in St Kitt's and led an anti-slavery campaign in the mid 19th century[14] By the same token we know next to nothing of the work of Dr Mathie Hamilton in Peru,[15] of Henry and David Coats in Rio de Janeiro,[16] or of a host of other Scottish doctors who practised in that vast continent.

The present collection of papers is an important addition to our understanding of the Scottish outreach over the centuries, an expansion which recognised no geographical, cultural or racial boundaries. Although heavily weighted towards the imperial domains and the white dominions, Scottish medicine was never restricted solely to these regions. Given the current levels of activity of the Universities and the Royal Colleges, it seems likely that Medicine Furth of Scotland will continue to be an important element in the provision of health care world-wide.

The Medieval Traffic with Europe

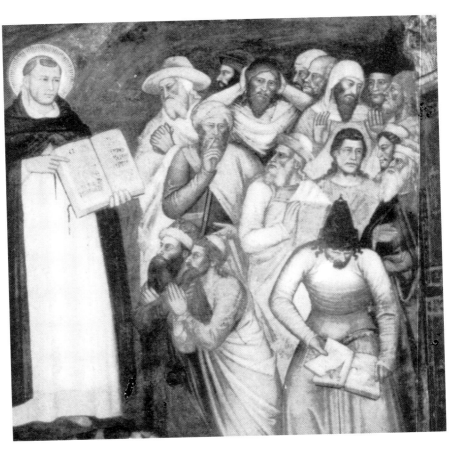

Michael Scot, the best-known Scottish medieval mediciner, kneeling centre-stage (in skull cap), in Gaddi's fresco of St Thomas Aquinas Converting Unbelievers, c.1330.

Chapter 1

The Medieval Traffic with Europe

J D Galbraith

'. . . on dit en proverbe
Que d'Escossois, de rats, de poux
Ceux qui voyagent jusqu'au bout
Du monde, en rencontrent partout . . .'

'The Scot goes to Bruges, and strolls the streets . . .'

That there was an intimate connection between Scotland and the
Continent in the later Middle Ages is too well known to require
further amplification here, apart perhaps from the (still necessary)
caution that the 'Auld Alliance' of 1295 was not the only such link,
or even the most obviously fruitful. However, this traffic had no
recognisable effect on the development of medical science in the years
before 1500.[1]

We might be justified in imagining that the alleged founder of the
first faculty of medicine in the British Isles would not have agreed
with this verdict.[2] Besides being a diplomat, canon lawyer, founder of
what might arguably be called the last of the 'medieval universities'
and bishop of the rather extensive diocese of Aberdeen, William
Elphinstone (1431-1514) 'gaderit', or more probably caused to be
gathered, legends of the saints of 'Scotland' which had not been
systematically placed in the order of worship of the Scottish church
before his time. The resulting compilation demonstrates that the
Scottish clergy of the early 16th century believed that the Scots had
received the gospel at an early date, and had exercised an influence
on their neighbours which was quite out of proportion to the size of
their country.[3] Certainly, the arrival of St Columba at Iona in 563
marked the beginning of a missionary enterprise of astonishing scale,
which apparently brought some medical knowledge in its train.

Columba himself was of course a noted worker of miracles, and not only in his own lifetime:

> 'On the following day he (Bishop George Brown of Dunkeld) blessed water, in which he dipped a bone of St Columba, and sent it . . . for the sick to drink. Many partook and were made whole. But one pert fellow answered the chancellor: "Why sends the bishop water for us to drink? I had rather he had sent to me the best of his ale". That man perished of the plague with the rest that did not receive the water of St Columba...'[4]

This incident reputedly took place in 1500, perhaps two to three years before Elphinstone's faculty of medicine at Aberdeen became fully effective.[5] It may give cause for some speculations on the state of medicine in Scotland at that time, besides testifying to Columba's reputation as a thaumaturge. But such extraordinary persons are not normally called upon to cure nose-bleeds, even very persistent ones,[6] so that Columba and his followers quite possibly derived much of their reputation as healers from the use of more conventional methods. In this respect, it is interesting to note that Columba was associated in Highland tradition with St John's wort, believed to be a particularly efficacious remedy.[7] It is known that St Gall in Switzerland, one of the most important 'Scottish' foundations on the Continent, had a noted physic garden, and given the influence exercised on learning in Anglo-Saxon England by another such foundation, Lindisfarne, it is hardly surprising to find 'Scottish' cures and charms in a Saxon leechdom.[8] Charms associated with the 'Celtic' saints seem to have been widespread and persistent. Columba's aid is called for in a German charm of the 14th century, for much the same reason as he was invoked in Highland charms.[9] The author of the celebrated *Breviarium Practice* (generally attributed to Arnald de Villanova and to the 13th century) cites an *experimentum* tried out by Master H[enry] the Englishman to treat the bite of a serpent or viper, which involved the use of holy water, a charm, and what looks like a prayer in standard form, beginning:

> 'Lord, Who by Thy marvellous power gave the blessed Brandan, Thy confessor, the virtue of expelling venom, . . .'

Arnald felt reluctantly obliged to include this '*obscenum*' because he had stated at the start of his work that he wished to 'bring together all the *experiments* of the principal doctors'.[10]

However, despite the fact that the Scottish clergy appropriated St Columba and other 'Celtic' saints for their own, these, and the 'herd of philosophers' who flocked to the Continent in the 9th century, were Scots from Ireland.[11] In general, no clear distinctions are made between the Scots of Erin and those of Alba until the 13th century. Apart from the episode of the crusades, these other Scots first become recognisable in Europe as scholars at the *studia generalia* which had developed in the century before.[12] One of the most celebrated of these early scholars in the sphere of 'philosophy' was Master (as he always seems to be styled) Michael Scot.[13]

Scot's present doubtful reputation seems to have been almost entirely the creation of his own countrymen (assuming that he was in fact Scottish).[14] The same could be said of many of the generally accepted facts concerning his early life. Another 'wizard', also called Scott, and his contemporary, James Hogg, were, as might be expected, particularly prominent among the inventors of 'Sir' Michael Scot of Balwearie, the warlock who split the Eildon Hills in three, held a contest in magic with Roger Bacon, and flew to Rome with snow on his hat.[15] Perhaps the only really remarkable thing about these, and similarly entertaining legends, is that they did not begin in Scot's own lifetime, or even (with one exception) immediately thereafter.

The first proven date in Michael Scot's career is 1217, when he was a translator at Toledo, a centre of study which his contemporaries associated with dubious activities:

> 'In Paris the scholars seek the arts, in Orleans the authors, in Bologna codices, in Salerno gallipots, in Toledo demons — and nowhere good manners'.[16]

Moreover, about three years later, Scot entered the service of the Emperor Frederick II, and began an apparently close association with him.17 It is perhaps worth a slight digression to summarise the '*stupor*' which Frederick inspired, and the place which some observers thought he occupied in the world picture, at least after his excommunication in 1227; for this purpose no-one could be more suitable than Salimbene de Adam (1221-c.1288), who had once been, on his own admission, an admirer of Frederick.[18] Witness, the account he gives of how he had learned of the Emperor's death:

> 'I myself could scarcely believe that he was dead . . . until I heard it with my own ears from the mouth of Pope Innocent IV, when he preached in the midst of the people at Ferrara...For I was so close to him that I could touch him (*semper eum tangebam*) when he said in his preaching "That emperor, our adversary, and the foe of God and his Church, had ended his life, as has been surely reported to us" I was astonished when I heard it, and could hardly believe it. For I was a follower of Joachim, and believed, and expected, and hoped that

Frederick would do many more evils than he had done, although he had done
many (*quamvis multa fecisset*)[19]

Neither his association with the diabolic rites of 'Salamanca's cave',[20] nor with Brother Salimbene's disappointingly abortive Antichrist, seems to have reflected noticably on Scot's personal reputation during the centuries when his works were current — and his *Liber physonomie* went through several editions from the 1470s, when the art of printing extended to this type of material — with the exception of Dante, who places Scot in Hell, perhaps, as always, for political rather than moral reasons.[21] But we are not lacking in contemporary assessments of Scot: he was a prophet (according to Salimbene, who classes him with Joachim of Fiore, Merlin, the Sybyll, St Methodius, Isaiah, Jeremiah, Hosea, Daniel, and the author of the Apocalypse, which is pretty respectable company, for the most part);[22] a scholar 'who flourishes among other men of learning with a singular gift of science' (Pope Honorius III) and who was 'well learned, not only in Latin, but also in Hebrew and the Arabic tongue' (Pope Gregory IX);[23] a 'true astrologer' (Salimbene again, this time quoting the presumed opinion given by Frederick II when Scot had computed the distance between the top of a palace and the heavens, and discovered a discrepancy in a similar calculation he had made some months earlier — Frederick had had the height of the buiding lowered in secret, while Scot was absent);[24] or a man, though in this case summed up with other of the writer's contemporaries, 'knowing neither sciences nor languages' (Roger Bacon).[25]

Evidently, Michael Scot was not without reputation in his own time, and, in the Middle Ages, such distinguished scholars were liable to have a variety of works and *experimenta* attributed to them; Frederick's Court, and those associated with it, attracted such attributions as easily as a jam-jar discarded on a summer's picnic attracts wasps.[26] One such attribution is that Michael Scot was actually a doctor by profession, and no less than Frederick's personal physician.[27] At least this is more respectable (though in the next three centuries, not yet wholly respectable) than the reputation foisted on him by writers of the 19th century.

Scot's reputation as a mediciner began fairly soon after his death in around 1236, if Arnald de Villanova (1235-1312) was indeed the author of the *Breviarium Practice*, in which this recipe is given:

'To provoke sleep so profound that a man may be cut and feel nothing, as if

> he were dead, and it is an *experimentum* of Master Michael Scott. Take opium
> thebacci (?), mandragora bark and henbane root . . . pound them together and
> mix with cold water . . . When you wish to sew or cut a man, dip a cloth
> in this and put it to his forehead . . . and nostrils, and he will swiftly sleep
> to deeply that you may do what you wish...'[28]

'*Experimentum*' rings authentically in this case, in that it accords with
the empirical approach sometimes evident in Scot's *Liber inroductorius*,
and very evident in his patron's treatise on the *Art of Hunting with Birds*,
which could still be recommended to bird-watchers of the present
century, since it is based on personal experience and observation.[29]
What is more, there is evidence that Frederick had a *curiositas* on the
subject of surgery, and we do not have to rely entirely on that same
genial Franciscan's word for it:

> 'He cut off a notary's thumb because he did not spell his [the Emperor's] name
> how he wished, for he wished that he should spell his name 'Fridericus' and he
> spelled it 'Fredericus . . .'
>
> '. . . He fed two men most excellently at dinner, of which one he sent to sleep
> and the other to hunt, and the next evening had them disembowelled in his
> presence, because he wished to know who had digested better. And it was
> judged by the physicians that he who had slept had enjoyed the best digestion
> . . .'[30]

However, it is curious that Salimbene does not associate Scot with
this, almost the most bizarre example of Frederick's *superstitiones* which
he reports, particularly since Scot is the principal character in the next
(measuring the distance between the heavens and tops of buildings). To
judge by Scot's own works, he had some knowledge of surgery, though
gained by observation rather than practice.[31] His one piece of advice
to Frederick on the subject (though it must be admitted that he uses
the word *consilium* in the sense of advice to a patient at an early date)
appears to have been given on the occasion when he warned the
Emperor against blood-letting in Gemini, since, during that sign, there
was danger of a second cut being made. (Frederick's barber disputed
this, made a successful incision, and then, no doubt in an extravagant
gesture of triumph, dropped his lancet on the Emperor's foot).[32]
In short, there seems to be no justifiable cause for thinking that
Arnald's experimentum is anything more than another of the medieval
spongia somnifera (doubtful as to efficacy, if not always as to
attribution), which has been hung on Scot's name to give the repute
of the compound greater weight.[33] The various pills and powders
ascribed to Scot have also been credited to him without clear cause.[34]
Scot apparently did know something of medicine, as indeed his works

reveal that he knew something of alchemy and of music. At the same
time, the *Liber phsionomie* and the tract *De urinis* incorporated therein,
are the only works touching on medicine which can be clearly
identified as his, albeit there are some indications that he had observed,
and even treated diseases.[35] But there is no substantial evidence that
he was a physician by profession, or even that he had been formally
trained in medicine.

Perhaps the story of Frederick's blood-letting provides some clue
about Scot's approach to this branch of science. The bulk of the
available evidence suggests that he was primarily interested in
astrology, and particularly in its practical applications, among which,
medicine was one of the most obvious and beneficial to humanity.
Roger Bacon would have agreed, in this instance, with Scot's
approach:

> '. . . the whole of medical practice is based on the study of atmospheric changes
> due to the influence of the spheres and stars. Wherefore a physician who knows
> not how to take into account the positions and aspects of the planets can effect
> nothing in the healing arts except by chance and good fortune. This is taught
> by . . . Hippocrates, Galen, Constantine, Rhazes, Haly, . . .'[36]

How far Michael was influenced by such authorities (as Bacon
evidently was), and whether he in turn influenced the physician/
astrologers of the later Middle Ages, are questions which may be
worthy of some further study. We might also wonder whether the
majority of the happy ignoramuses who actually practised medicine
took any notice at all, considering that Paracelsus (1493-1541) can still
be found shouting the same message as Bacon almost three centuries
later. Thus we might fairly conclude that Michael Scot made a
recognisable contribution to learning in the Middle Ages as a
translator, particularly of Aristotle's *De Animalibus*, but that he had no
tangible influence on the development of medicine.

The same can be said of the Scots who studied medicine in Europe
during the 14th and 15th centuries. Of course, Bernard Gordon,
teacher at Montpellier, author of the *Lilium Medicinae* (1303), and,
according to Chaucer, one of the most eminent physicians of his day,
has been claimed as Scottish; this, as well as claims to French or
English nationality, remains unproven.[37] William Baillie, who lectured
at Ferrara in the mid 15th century, seems to have passed into
obscurity, together with his two medical treatises.[38] Reflection on the
19th century tradition of 'the Enterprising Scot' may make this lack
of initiative in the medicine of an earlier period seem curiously out

of character, erroneous, or downright disappointing. It should not, if we pause to consider something of the circumstances in which medicine was taught and practised, and the particular circumstances of the Scottish students themselves.

The scholarly world of the later Middle Ages had one singular advantage over that even of the present century — communication: everyone in that itinerant world of study spoke, wrote, disputed, heard lectures and went to worship (where they would no doubt hear more than the occasional sermon on students' excesses), in the same language. The medieval student also had one suitable disadvantage compared with his modern counterpart — communication. To paraphrase Messrs Sellar and Yeatman: the medieval disciplines of arts and medicine were not what you thought, they were (largely) what you could remember.[39] This rather obvious point deserves to be laboured in order to emphasise that, in an age when books, and even materials for note-taking, were expensive, it was natural that teaching methods should have been designed above all to reinforce instruction at every stage. Thus the student might typically spend a substantial part of his second year listening again to the material covered in his first, and so throughout the course; also, on the basis that he would remember facts more clearly if he had thought them out (or dressed them up) for himself, an integral part of his curriculum would be to dispute various propositions with his fellows, formally as well as informally.[40] Medicine, like the other higher studies (law and theology) was taught in this fashion, as a discipline based on a set course of lectures dealing with a limited number of standard authorities. This course had been fixed as early as Michael Scot's day; a *corpus* of short texts called the *Articella*, compiled mainly from the works of Hippocrates and Galen, which, with the later addition of texts from Arabian sources, formed the basis of instruction throughout the Middle Ages. It was of course merely the basis, on which was built a whole structure of microscopic analysis, involved commentary and intense disputation on matters of detail: but the 'philosophical' physicians of the universities would no more have questioned the essential validity or sufficiency of their authorities than the theologians would have questioned the authority of scripture, or wished to improve on it, albeit both were quite ready to engage in involved debate on the interpretation of individual words. One gets the distinct impression that the subject taught was secondary to the purpose of the discipline — any of the disciplines — which was to teach the recollection, analysis, and presentation of facts; in short, how to 'think'. But medicine could never quite be forced into the mould of the other disciplines — there was an awkward side to it called 'practice', for which provision was made in the curriculum.[41] It seems appropriate to say something of the medieval books of practice at this point.

The other two higher disciplines were 'practical' also, of course, and although this is least obvious in the case of divinity, that discipline provides the most illuminating parallel with the works of the practitioners, or '*medici*'.[42] Divinity in action is preaching, which was given an impetus by the Fourth Lateran Council of 1215, at which bishops were urged to licence sufficient preachers in their dioceses.[43] 'Handbooks' (wanting a better word) for preachers became part of the literature of Europe. These are generally arranged by topics which might constitute the subject of a sermon; a further refinement was to arrange these subjects alphabetically from, say '*Abstinencia*' to '*Ypocrisis*'.[44] Under each of the several headings, whether dealing with the virtues of temperance, or the dreadful fate of hypocrites, could usually be found relevant quotes from scripture, the Doctors of the Church, saint's legends, and on occasion, the author's personal stamp; relevant 'examples' which he had used himself or had picked up, the inclusion of which would swell the body of sermon-making literature. Such a compendium might then be (typically) called 'A little Handfull of Flowers' or something of the sort: this form of title, in itself, might arouse curiosity as to the nature and composition of contemporary medical treatises bearing titles like 'The English Rose' or 'The Lily of Medicine', both of which, incidentally, were of great repute.[45] On closer acquaintance, it indeed appears that these 'practical' works of the mediciners are similar to those of the preachers; they are arranged by 'conditions' (physical rather than moral), for each of which we might find some combination of the unquestioned dictates of ancient authority, the statements and nostrums of lesser and more recent authorities, recalled from teaching or culled from books, and accounts of the writer's own experiences in giving treatment, coupled with others he had learned from his fellows; like those cited by Arnald de Villanova, something of whose *experimenta* we have already seen:

> '. . . an *experimentum* which I had from Brother John . . .'
> '. . . a certain Frenchman told me that . . .'
> '. . .Master Hector of England swore to me that he had cured many
> . . . with this unction . . .'[46]

Presumably, armed with your *Flos*, *Breviarium* or *Theatrum*, you could (provided that you had recognised the patient's complaint with some degree of accuracy) have recourse to a variety of possible treatments, using the next when the first had failed, until the patient either recovered, or was no longer in a position to co-operate. (Perish the though that this did not necessarily mean that he was dead).

In the light of this brief (and very generalised) summary of the teaching and practice of medicine in the Middle Ages, it would be convenient to conclude that the Scots made no contribution to the development of medical science because nobody else did. To do this, unfortunately, would be to give an incomplete picture on both counts. Medical knowledge had increased by the late Middle Ages, and, given the constraints of the period, we might go so far as to assess this development as substantial — it even included something akin to plastic surgery;[47] also the lack of Scottish involvement in medicine might be largely a consequence of these constraints, albeit coupled with other possible factors.

The basic similarity of approach to 'practical' theology and to 'practical' medicine may imply that the latter was virtually static, but does not mean that it was wholly respectable. The Lateran Council of 1215 while encouraging the one, disadvantaged the other, in that clerics in major orders were forbidden to shed blood, which stricture specifically prohibited them from the practice of surgery (unless, to give the canon the widest possible interpretation, this art could be studied without the need to make incisions.)[48] So surgery continued to be taught and studied, though in a rather informal 'come as you please' atmosphere outwith the university curriculum[49] — this at least involved some kind of practical experience in that students were generally taken to hospitals to watch, thereby acquiring, no doubt, one or two common-sense rules that are still valid:

> '. . . one of the students fainted as soon as he saw the brain pulsating. So my
> advice is that no-one should undertake an operation until he has first seen it
> performed . . .'[50]

Surgery was not respectable; moreover its practice, and that of 'practical' medicine in general, was largely in the hands of barber-surgeons, leeches and other practitioners of folk-remedies, and similarly unlettered persons with no grounding in the arts or any licence to practise from an established school of medicine. It is scarcely surprising that the physicians of the universities stressed the 'philosophical' aspect of medicine rather than any practical element, since they were forced to defend their dignity and privileges against the unlicensed rabble of practitioners on one side, and on the other, the lawyers, who could cite such people as evidence that medicine was no more than a mechanic art, not worthy to be ranked with the study of law.[51] Thus practice, whether in or outwith the university environment, was, as described earlier, an 'awkward' element in medicine, in that it diminished the status of that study as a true discipline. We might sum all this up by concluding that medicine was the least prestigious of the higher degrees, and turn at last to consider how Scottish students might have approached it.

Students of the 14th and 15th centuries were not as obviously altruistic as some of their counterparts in the 12th century; would any of them have gone, like Gerard of Cremona, to Toledo purely out of love of Ptolomy's *Almagest*, because he could not find it in Latin?[52] In the later Middle Ages, where you took your degree, and in what, often mattered a great deal; the Scots were probably no exception to this career-conscious attitude to study.[53] They had a particular problem of their own — that there was an expensive and sometimes dangerous journey to be made before they began their studies.[54]

From then on, the Scottish student would merely have to cope with the same expenses as his fellows, of whatever country, and these could be considerable; besides maintaining himself and paying his fees, he would have to contribute his share to various 'festivities', provide a feast when he graduated, and be prepared to incur yet further cost when, or if, he assumed academic office.[55] But to judge by the records of Paris University (which are fortunately very complete, since this was the resort, at least initially, of most Scots), few students were exempted from payment of the regular 'quot' because they were poor.[56] There was, of course, the occasional exception[57] and one notorious deception (perhaps presuming on a reputation Scotland had already acquired as a poor country):

> '. . . John Kennedy . . . had his means assessed (*fecit–taxari bursas–suas*) by Master Henry de Merxem, then procurator, at 4 *solidos*, in the guise (*specie*) of a pauper. The nation [was] credibly informed that he was kin to the greatest of the kingdom of Scotland, nephew of a certain bishop [James Kennedy of St Andrews], and richly beneficed, since he was provost of a certain venerable church in Scotland [Maybole]; item, he had brought with him at his coming to Paris a good 100 crowns, and had received thereafter 50 crowns and 20 nobles...'[58]

Master Kennedy, 'not wishing to deceive the nation' then offered to pay ten crowns, but was still threatened with expulsion. His case is worth quoting because it emphasises that only a small proportion of the population of Scotland could afford an education on the Continent, and that those who could required a substantial income, either from private means or funding, or, as in Kennedy's case, from the revenue of a benefice; perhaps it is as true as most generalities to say that one of the objects of study for those who did not already have a benefice was to obtain one.[59]

It is difficult to see what attractions the study of medicine would have had for such men, though a few took it — in some cases perhaps from simple curiosity. The proven way to advancement was by studying law; canon law at Paris and, since career opportunities in this field fluctuated, preferably also civil law at Orleans, to attain, ideally, the status of a doctor *utriusque juris*. By contrast, all that the pursuit of medicine had to offer was the acquisition of knowledge beneficial (in theory at least) to mankind — though there is not enough evidence for this period to suggest how far it was studied for that reason, if at all — and the blandishments of the *medici*, which are of a part with other available evidence on the motivation of medieval doctors:

> '. . . believe me, whoever wishes honour, riches, glory, thanks of men, let him pay heed to this book . . .'[60]

> '. . . it is a special secret of my own which should neither be prepared or taught to anyone but on first receiving the price of treatment, for it cures within a short space . . .'[61]

Chaucer, naturally, had noticed something of the sort:

> '. . . gold in phisik is a cordial,
> Therefore he lovede gold in special'[62]

Unfortunately, those who, like many Scots, derived their funds for study from a benefice, were debarred from the attractions of heaping up gold, if not from the chance of being 'eternised for some wondrous cure'. There were occasional salutary examples of what happened to beneficed men who practised medicine for profit 'to the opprobrium of the clerical state'.[63]

Whatever the reasons, few Scots studied medicine, out of the very small proportion of Scots who studied any higher discipline at all, and, as Scottish graduates generally returned to Scotland after completing their studies, it would indeed be remarkable if the inhabitants of that small country, 'beyond which there is no dwelling place at all'[64] had made any tangible contribution to the development of the science.

But the word 'traffic' implies movement in more than one direction.

Medicine on the Continent certainly influenced Scottish practice. Given that comparatively few medieval manuscripts of any sort have survived in this country, it is interesting to find some medical texts among the survivors, besides occasional hints of others which have perished.[65] From the later 15th century, when printed books were regularly imported into Scotland, the intimacy of this traffic becomes very evident. Scotland faced the same medical problems as the rest of Europe, although there is no real evidence to suggest that the Scots of this period chose to interpret the reason for recurrent plagues, and particularly for a 'new' one (actually an old one, awareness of which had been spread by printing) in the same fatalistic way as some of their neighbours in northern Europe — as yet further evidence of the coming dissolution of the world at or around the half-millenium of 1500:

> '. . . As the result of such sins, formerly famine and earthquakes and pestilence
> . . . fell on the earth, and still [remain] in our days, moreover, that new and
> most grave *morbus* of men, risen in our days, which is vulgarly called the *Malum*
> *Francicum*, never heard of before . . . [66]

In general, the earliest printed works on syphilis, dating from 1497-8, ascribe its cause to the wrath of God, or the influence of the stars, and propose mercurial salves as a cure, on the assumption that it was a mere skin disease. Hans Widmann of Tubingen, writing in 1497, is rather out of the ordinary, in that he recommended avoidance of intercourse with infected women or prostitutes: in this context it is worth remarking that one later writer, at least, denied that the disease was sexually transmitted.[67] Widmann, of course, had specialised in the treatment of leprosy, and his recommended measures had been found effective in the containment of that disease. However, given the contemporary conflict of opinion on how to approach treatment of the 'malady of France', it is curious that two Scottish burghs took positive action of the sort enjoined by Widmann, in the same year as his treatise was published; of all Scottish burghs these two apparently had the closest links with northern Europe. The council of Aberdeen regulated against promiscuity.[68] That of Edinburgh quarantined sufferers, and those treating them, on the island of Inchkeith, which would have amounted to the same thing for practical purposes, of course.[69] Perhaps all that this proves, though, is that Scottish burghs knew as much as Continental cities about how to deal with leprosy and the plague.

Edinburgh's decision to quarantine was in fact instigated by King

James IV, who was interested in medicine, as in many other things. According to Robert Lindsay of Pitscottie, he used Inchkeith for another purpose:

> '. . . he wished to experiment regarding what language and speech children would have while growing, if no-one spoke to them. And so he ordered the foster-mothers and nurses . . . on no account to prattle or speak to them. For he wished to know whether they would acquire the Hebrew language, which was the first, or Greek, or Latin, or Arabic, or the particular language of their parents. But . . . the children all died, because they could not live without hand-claps and face-making and smiles and blandishments from the nurses . . .'[70]

Intriguingly, this is not Pitscottie, but Salimbene's account of one of Frederick II's *curiositates* which went wrong. The two instances as reported are remarkably similar, except that James did rather better. He introduced the refinement of ensuring that the nurses were deaf and dumb; presumably they could then play with the children without the risk of compromising their mission, and, if we are to believe Pitscottie, the youngsters ended up speaking 'good Hebrew' (or so he had heard).[71] Even in late medieval Scotland, the spirit of *experimentum* was clearly not yet dead.

The Scots and Military Medicine

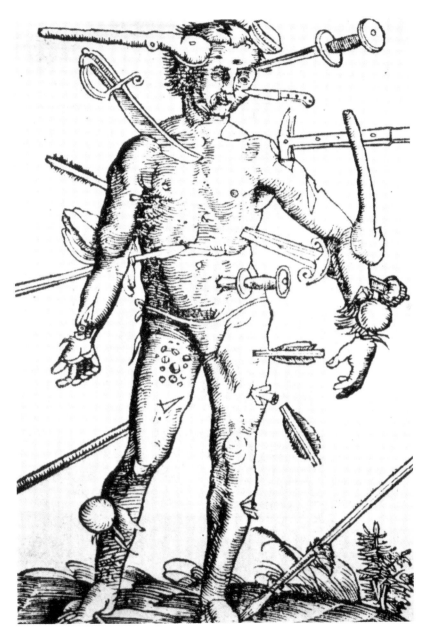

The 'wound man' of Paracelsus, 1536. Cold steel would soon be replaced by gunshot wounds as the primary worry of the military doctor.

Chapter 2
The Scots and Military Medicine
J S G Blair

Military medicine has formed an important branch of the profession since time immemorial, largely as a result of mankind's inclination towards armed conflict in the pursuit of power or territorial expansion. The nature of the work of the military surgeon began to change in the late medieval period with the application of gunpowder to the propulsion of missiles, a development which may have seemed as terrifying to contemporary soldiers as the nuclear bomb is in our own time. Whether it was the Englishman Roger Bacon in the 13th century, or the German monk Bernard Schwartz in the 14th who actually invented gunpowder,[1] it was not until the siege of Parma in the 16th that musketeers first proved their worth.

Although De Vigo in 1514 was the first to use the term 'gunshot wound', it was during the service of the great Ambrois Paré, between the battle of Turin in 1536 and the battle of Moncontour in 1569, that the term was used regularly. The later more detached descriptions of John Hunter in 1794 are so often quoted by British medical historians, but they do not convey the realities of battlefield wounding as do the earlier writings of Paré. He described head and chest injuries, but his most striking accounts are of wounds of the limbs. He describes the ball shattering the wrist, arm or foot, the amputation, the staunching of blood by the hot iron, the subsequent tetanus with death or recovery, the compound fracture of the femur with osteomyelitis lasting many months, the pieces of dirty uniform or soil carried into the body by the missile. He describes the certainty of death in abdominal wounds — though notes how recovery can take place if a colostomy is formed and provides natural drainage. He describes the 'terrible dyspnoea, sense of suffocation, insupportable anxiety and faintness' associated with penetrating wounds of the chest. Paré's use of bland dressings for amputation stumps instead of the terrible cautery was only one of the great advances in military surgery introduced by the man who is arguably the greatest war surgeon of all time.

In the later 16th century the continued universal use of Latin provided a European dimension still not recovered in our own time, and attracted some Scottish doctors into the service of the super-powers of the day, Spain and France. Probably the best known of these was Maister Peter Lowe, founder of the Faculty of Physicians and Surgeons of Glasgow in 1599, who served both sides as a surgeon during the previous decade.[2] The emergence of Britain as a major sea power after the Union of 1603, and the establishment of a colonial presence in the Americas and the East Indies, created opportunities for naval and army medical service in an ever-widening range of overseas territories. Much of this expansion was, inevitably, accompanied by armed conflict and new challenges for military doctors.

Pain was the symptom above all others in war wounds of these centuries which emerges from all good accounts as terrifying in its degree and its continuance.[3] Infection was the almost universal sequel to wounding in later days or weeks. Infection in the form of gastrointestinal, skin, or epidemic diseases was the great destroyer of armies in the period of static camp, marches, or garrison duty, and to infection was added, as far as the Royal Navy was concerned, deficiency diseases from malnutrition while on long sea voyages. And as European navies and armies began to campaign in the tropics, the whole spectrum of tropical disease was added to those found in a temperate climate. It has of course to be remembered that diseases regarded today as purely tropical — malaria and cholera are examples — were in these centuries found widely over Europe.

Scotsmen made a major contribution to military surgery and medicine from the 17th century onwards. Those involved over the centuries since the formation of a standing army can be divided into three groups: the medical innovators, the medical administrators, and the rank and file medical officers. It is fair to say that the third group produced as great persons as the first and second. The Royal Navy is the first of our Services, as every honest soldier and airman will admit. It also led the way in medical care, initially under the guidance of King Charles I, a Scotsman, who pursued improved conditions for sailors by instituting a formal system of hospital ships, a free allowance of drugs and postgraduate lectures in the specialty of naval medicine within the Company of Barber Surgeons in London. The best remembered of these lecturers was Alexander Reid (1586-1641), an Aberdeen graduate. And it was Charles II, at the Restoration in 1660, who — amongst other changes connected with the establishment of the reduced standing army — had commissioned medical officers appointed on a regular basis.

It is a truth that famous men are not necessarily good men and not necessarily even able or clever. William Cockburn (Edinburgh and Leyden) was such a one. Well-born, influential, and very confident, he joined the Fleet in 1694 and at the age of 26 wrote a book on Sailors' Diseases which became a standard work in two years. Later he became an MD and FRS, and is to date the only naval physician to be buried in Westminster Abbey. But he was not original, not an attractive character, and his views were out of date even when he wrote them. He prescribed lemon juice for scurvy, but drew no conclusion from its success. We have all met his type. But James Lind was a man of true greatness. Born in Edinburgh, apprenticed to a doctor there at the age of 15, he entered the Navy as a surgeon's mate in 1739. (This was the same year that Smollet joined.) By 1747 Lind was surgeon of HMS *Salisbury*, a 60-gun ship, on which he made his epoch-making experiment on scurvy, the first controlled dietary experiment in the history of medicine. In 1748 he took his MD at Edinburgh, his dissertation being *De Morbis Veneris Localibus*. His *Dissertation on Fevers and Infections* published in 1761, some years after he had left the Service, entitles him to be regarded as the 'Father of Preventive Medicine'. It begins: 'The number of seamen in time of war who die by shipwreck, capture, famine, fire or sword are but inconsiderable in respect of such as are destroyed by the ship diseases and by the usual maladies of intemperate climates'.

In 1758 Lind was appointed senior physician to Haslar Hospital, where he remained till 1783. The sudden deterioration in naval standards within a few years of his departure may seem hard to credit after a man of Lind's greatness had been in charge, but it is a sequence of events all too commonly repeated in British military history. Smollet in *Roderick Random* described the horrors of the Navy and naval medicine in the 18th century — the perfunctory training of ships' surgeons, the appalling squalor of the sick bay, the brutality of the prototype Captain Oakum. Scots were prominent in reform of the medical branch — Thomas Trotter of Edinburgh from 1790, whose *Medicina Nautica* of 1796 was the precursor of the *Journal of the Royal*

Naval Medical Service, and Gilbert Blane, from Ayrshire and Glasgow. He, like Trotter, was a medical *administrator* rather than a clinical innovator. He was an inspirer of the divisional system in the Royal Navy, an early proponent of the truth that health depends as much upon the executive officers as upon the medical officers. His words on this point were quoted unchanged by the Naval Director-General in the Second World War. The Blane medal, for meritorious service by a naval surgeon, is named after him.

These men were officers in the medical service of the Royal Navy. Lind had a counterpart of equal greatness in the Army, and he too was a Scot. Sir John Pringle was born in 1707 at Stitchel. He started his medical career at St Andrews, where Simson *primus* had begun lectures as the first Chandos professor in 1721. He moved to Edinburgh in 1727, to study further, but left within a year for Leyden. According to James Boswell, Pringle intended on leaving Scotland to follow a mercantile career, but after hearing a lecture by the now elderly Boerhaave, decided on a medical career after all. Returning to Scotland he entered clinical practice, but joined the Army medical service of the day and by the good offices of Lord Stair, its commander-in-chief, was appointed physician to the Army in Flanders in 1742 and Physician-General in 1745. During his six years in Flanders, where the British Army had 28,000 men at its maximum, he established the Scottish connection with British and Continental military medicine, via Edinburgh and Leyden. His great innovations encompassed both administration and epidemiology. It was due to his efforts that military hospitals were first recognised as neutral territory and could be safely set up near a battlefield. At the battle of Dettingen in 1743, under a 'Temporary Red Cross', and with the agreement of the Duc de Noailles, the French commander, British and French hospitals were set up side by side, each taking wounded from the other army if the occasion arose. In this Pringle anticipated the Geneva Convention by 120 years.

Although Pringle left the Physician-General's post in 1748, he did not publish his *Observations on Diseases of the Army* till 1752. This watershed work has probably never received the credit it deserves in history, let alone in military history. Like Lind, Pringle had quickly recognised hospitals as, to use his own words, 'among the chief causes of sickness and death in the Army'. His special contribution was the first scientific account of epidemiology, prevention of cross-infection, and, it can be argued, of antiseptics. Criticisms made of Pringle by some are invalid, if the progress of his thought is followed carefully. Let us hear his own words, as expressed in the fourth edition of his *Observations*:

> '. . . in the camp, the contagion (of dysentery) passes from one who is ill to his companions in the same tent, and from them perhaps to the next. The foul straw becomes very infectious. But of what nature is this infection? In the former editions of this work, I considered the spreading of the distemper as owing to putrid exhalations of the humours of those who first fell ill of it; and that when this *miasma* is received into the blood, I conceived it to act upon the whole mass as a ferment, disposing it to putrefaction . . . But having since perused the curious dissertation, published by *Linnaeus*, in favour of *Kircher's* system of contagion by *animalcula*, it seems reasonable to suspend all *hypotheses*, till the matter is further enquired into'.

In his thinking he was influenced by the great men of Leyden:

> 'Leeuwenhoeck had shown "small insects" in the pustules of scabies, under the microscope . . . So the frequency of the itch is not to be ascribed to change of air or diet, but to the infection propagated by a few such . . .'

Pringle's consideration of the possibility of microscopic contamination then led him to think in terms of 'septic' and 'antiseptic':

> 'The faeces are rendered less, if at all infectious, by means of a strong acid combined with the parts that are really septic — especially, in the dysentery, where the faeces are highly corrupted and contagious . . .'

He even considered the systemic use of such 'antiseptics':

> 'were putrefaction the only change made in the body by contagion, it would be easy to cure such fevers, at any period, by the use of acids, or other antiseptics'.

Yet Pringle is not mentioned by Dr WAR Thomson in his *History of Antisepsis* (1963) and it is almost certain that Lister knew nothing of his work.

John Hunter cannot be omitted in any record of Scots who contributed to military medicine. His *Treatise on the Blood, Inflammation and Gunshot Wounds* (1794), published the year after his death, contrasts with the work of these others in being the detached observations of the pathologist rather than the anxious involvement of the regimental medical officer. He saw the difference between gunshot and 'accidental' wounds as Paré did, noting the contamination of clothing, the effect of differing velocity and the 'strange course' of some balls in the former. Although surgeon to Bellisle in 1761 and Surgeon-General to the Army in 1790, he was less involved than Lind or Pringle in the care of the servicemen which was the special greatness of those two. Hunter's contributions must therefore be ranked somewhat lower in the scale.

Lack of involvement certainly cannot be ascribed to the next great man, Sir James McGrigor. Primarily an administrator, he had the rare gift of selecting colleagues whose own abilities he recognised and whose careers he supported for unselfish reasons. His most active years included the period of the wars with France from 1793-1814, and of colonial expansion, when military medicine was becoming an area of specialisation and service medical officers were learning clinical techniques, hospital administration, and sanitary codes more and more applicable to the rank and file and the lower deck.

James McGrigor was born in 1771 in Inverness-shire, attended school and university in Aberdeen, and graduated MA at Marischal College, one of the two adjacent universities in Aberdeen, in 1788. The formal study of medicine was not then possible at Aberdeen, so he became apprenticed to a physician who held an appointment in the Aberdeen Royal Infirmary, and began his career by washing bottles and instruments and preparing pills. He stayed briefly in Edinburgh but took no degree. He went to England in 1793, becoming assistant to a practitioner in Islington, then a village a mile and a half from London. Next, still without bothering to take a medical degree, he bought a commission for £150 in the newly formed 88th of Foot, the Connaught Rangers, on 25 September 1793.

As so often happens, the reforms of his predecessor Pringle had been quickly forgotten. McGrigor's career is so long and important that it is hard to describe shortly. He was influenced in his early years by Donald Monro, another Scottish graduate (from Edinburgh) as well as by Sir John Pringle's writings. Serving first in Flanders, then in the West and East Indies where he learned the effect of climate and tropical disease, he was an administrator of hospitals rather than a clinician. In the Peninsula he rose to high position, winning praise from Wellington for his casualty evacuation after Corunna, and becoming Inspector of Hospitals in 1809. At home, he fought the patronage of the haughty London-trained individuals in the Medical Board — Sir Lucas Pepys the Physician-General and Thomas Keate the Surgeon-General had society practices in London but had never served overseas. They feuded with Knight, the Inspector-General of Hospitals, who at least had. After defying his superiors during the expedition to the Scheldt and the disaster of Walcheren, McGrigor had a new Medical Board appointed, consisting of Dr John Weir of Aberdeen and

Dr Charles Ker of Edinburgh. Because war surgery was so grim, it attracted few cultivated, high quality men. McGrigor supported George James Guthrie, the most famous Army surgeon of the era, appreciating his abilities, and ensured his promotion. McGrigor's main claim to permanent fame was his skill in organising the removal of wounded. His process is still taught to our medical officers — how many of us realised, when we watched the training film 'The Way Back', that it was based on McGrigor's principles? The poor relief of casualties after Waterloo saddened him deeply, as did the lack of gratitude shown by the military establishment towards the common soldier and indeed towards the junior officer. He presided over the Medical Department for thirty-six years, assisted by one principal secretary till 1833 and then by a secretary and six clerks. His major reforms were:

1. The education of medical officers, after their selection. He personally screened applicants.

2. The development of Chairs of Military Medicine at Dublin and Edinburgh.

3. Assistance to widows and dependents.

4. Research into all aspects of army health.

5. Statistics — perhaps as important as any.

6. Royal Commissions for medical officers.

His statue broods over the RAMC Headquarters Mess garden at Millbank, of which all members of that Corps are so proud, and his spirit still pervades the corridors within. Nor has his Alma Mater forgotten him.

A near contemporary of McGrigor's also had an important role in the early 19th century European conflict. Sir James Wylie (1768-1854), from Kincardine-on-Forth was awarded the Aberdeen MD in 1794, and is recognised as the founder of Russian military medicine. He went to Russia in 1790 and in 1800 took the leading part in the foundation of the Department of Military Medicine in St Petersburg. He was Head of the Army Medical Department in Russia for twenty-five years, was physician and adviser to several Czars, and took a large part in the campaigns of 1812 and 1813. In 1968 Dr Norah Schuster published an article in the *Proceedings of the Royal Society of Medicine* entitled, most amusingly, '*English* Doctors in Russia in the early nineteenth century'.

Despite this title the only ones of distinction — Wylie, Sir Alexander Crichton, John Rogerson from Dumfries and Dr Robert Lyall - were all Scots!

The Indian Medical Service developed during the 19th century into a major institution of Empire, full of Scots' doctors from its earliest years. One of the first to gain distinction in this sphere was Simon Nicholson, a son of Kiltarlity manse in Inverness-shire. After training at St George's Hospital in London he travelled to Madras in 1802, and was 'possibly the best physician who ever practised in India.'[4] He was succeeded by Sir Ranald Martin from Skye, who was physician to the Secretary of State for India in the 1850s. Dirom Grey Crawford, the historian of the IMS, was an Edinburgh graduate who died in 1942 aged 85. Major-General Sir James Graham of Glasgow was DGIMS and Health Commissioner from 1924-33; he in turn was succeeded by Colonel Sir Alexander Russell, a St Andrews graduate who retired in 1939. The best-known of the IMS officers, however, was Sir Ronald Ross (1857-1932). His work on malaria established Ross as one of the greatest medical men of all time, yet he left India disgusted at the lack of appreciation shown to his monumental work. No formal thanks was ever made to him.

In additional these large-print names, Scotland produced men whose work at regimental level complemented the contributions of Lind, Pringle, McGrigor and Ross, and whose individual contributions earned them a reverence from their soldiers usually denied to the senior rank. They deserve an equal place in our history. The 18th century work of what we now call the RMO, the Regimental Medical Officer, could not be better described than by Robert Hamilton, whose *Duties of a Regimental Surgeon considered with observations on his General Qualifications, and hints relative to a MORE RESPECTABLE PRACTICE an a Better Regulation of that Department* (1787) takes as its preface 'More men die (in Regimental Practice) by the Lancet, than by the Lance'. This fascinating work covers the whole range of the RMO's work and the conditions of his service:

> 'Each Regiment, as well militia as regulars, is allowed a surgeon, as he is termed, and surgeon's mate. The surgeon is paid 4 shillings a day, the mate three and six, but as stoppages are levied from them of one shilling a day from the surgeon, and 6 pence from his mate, they make the same. The surgeon receives a commission signed by the Secretary at War, or, if abroad, by the Commander-in-Chief there, who has authority; the mate only a warrant signed by the Colonel of the Regiment he is to enter'.

Provision of billets, hiring of houses for the sick, local employment of nurses, conduct of the sick parade, attendance at field firing days ('to attend to any accident. Men cut their hands on the flints when firing, sometimes when returning their bayonets, or may collapse with fatigue') are all described, and practical instructions given. His comments on reduced establishments and restricted funding in peacetime have a contemporary ring.

The contents of the medical chest are an important chapter — lancets, an inhaler for use in throat inflammation, bed pans, bath tubs, bandages, leeches, ointments, catheters and syringes for gonorrhoea or wound sinuses are some of the items listed. The necessity of keeping high quality instruments in good condition is stressed. The carrying out of post mortem examinations by the RMO increases his surgical skill — 'cool, steady, deliberate intrepidity, where neither the heart shall fail nor the hands shake, is of all things the most requisite in this art'.

Hamilton is a shrewd analyst of the military environment. He notes the beneficent effect on the troops of a good Lieutenant-Colonel and good field officers. He is especially insistent on the care of families. He sees the need for reading medical journals — not only to keep himself up-to-date, but to maintain his status in the officers' mess. His practical advice for the RMO amongst his brother officers includes this classic sentence: 'The Regimental Surgeon should never be a drunkard — for he never knows when he may be called out: the other officers know when their duties are, and so can arrange things!'

A large and fascinating chapter of the book describes in great detail the duties in supervising military floggings. The tying of the delinquent to the halberds ought to be supervised to ensure that 'the arms must be tied above the wrists, not to put too great pressure on the hands . . . Cuts must not be risked elsewhere than on the back — not below the ribs, or the front or face. The Regimental Surgeon must see that the cats be small, so that they cut cleaner and bruise less (bruising the great fear). Should be changed soon because when soaked with blood they increase the severity of the stroke. Never punish after a March, nor field exercises, nor on the morning after a drunken debauch'. The RMO had by law the right to demand that a soldier be taken down, and 'the commanding officer has not it in his power to control him'. This in the late 18th century was a significant authority given to the doctor. In this as in all his comment and advice, Hamilton showed himself an unusually thoughtful and kindly officer.

Individual rank and file medical officers are so many that only a few can be recorded, to show the breadth of their contributions over the centuries. John McColme, Surgeon to the Royal Scots Regiment of Foot in Ireland, graduated MD at Aberdeen in October 1753; he 'sent in proper certificates and a solution of a case in Physick, with an aphorism of Hippocrates, had a regular education, and came off (the examination) with great applause' the Senate minute recorded.[5] In the first Afghan War of 1841, Assistant Surgeon Grant showed that the RMO could be an officer as well as a doctor: 'Mr. Grant — not the first MO who has played the part of the true soldier in battle, and justified the claims of his profession to the soldier's honours and rewards — having spiked the guns with his own hands, led out the main body, while Ensign Jones brought up the rear'. John Leyden, a Church of Scotland missionary and later MD St Andrews and MRCS Edinburgh, not only served with the Indian Medical Service but was a noted linguist, compiling grammars of Malay and Prakrit, and translating the gospels into five Indian languages.[6]

In the early years of the First World War a young bacteriologist from St Andrews, William John Tulloch, was posted to London to work on tetanus, which was claiming too many lives of the wounded in the agricultural soil of France. 'Tulloch types' remain the international standard classification of this organism to this day.

The Royal Air Force medical branch is a very new element in military medicine, but has already an established tradition in its own fields. Sir Charles Whittingham, a Glasgow graduate trained at that best of all pathology departments in the Kingdom between the Wars, was not only Director-General in the Second War but also initiated the RAF pathology service. He must be included in any list of outstanding Scots' contributions to military medicine.

Before the Second World War, the quiet highlanders DJ and FA Macrae came to St Andrews where Duncan was discovered to be one of the best centre three-quarters of the inter-war years. He was captured with the original Highland Division at St Valery. His younger brother Farquhar 'displayed remarkable coolness in evacuating many severely wounded officers and men' in the Alamein battle, was captured with his RAMC Sergeant, and quickly escaped. He was decorated for his bravery, and revered by his men in the 5th Seaforth battalion. Walter Yellowlees of the Edinburgh School was also decorated for bravery; his Camerons remembered him forever afterwards as *their* revered medical officer.[7]

But in the Second World War, the grimmest and cruellest

conditions endured by British and Commonwealth servicemen were those of the Japanese prisoners of war. George Blair, a St Andrews graduate of 1940, was RMO to camps in Formosa, now Taiwan. When he was ill with bacillary dysentery and his life hanging in the balance, hardened regular soldiers prayed for his recovery.[8] His birthday card, miraculously adorned with a sprig of heather, was signed by all 500 men in the camp. He, too, was decorated for gallantry as camp doctor. He kept his medical records hidden under the floor of his hospital, at the risk of his life. He presented these to the Royal Army Medical Corps Museum at Millbank thirty years after his release and before his death. He, too, received no note of acknowledgement from the curator of the day who was, sadly, another Scot — Major General Alastair MacLennan. His books of notes, recently re-discovered, have now provided clinical information for the current Professor of Medicine to use in his tropical medicine course. The Professor of Military Surgery commented: 'the extraordinary detail and neatness with which they were written under such dangerous conditions make them a tribute to what must have been a remarkable devotion on his part to the care of his patients'.

And so the past reaches the present, and its old notebooks are still of use to new medical officers. Let us end with two contemporary Scots who maintain the tradition of the centuries. The design for the new field operating table used by the Services is the brainchild of Colonel Frank McVicar of Glasgow, now returned to Arran as surgeon there. And since we began with an Aberdeen graduate, let us end with one — Brigadier Jack Coull, the outstanding surgeon presently serving in the RAMC, whose external fixation apparatus for lower limb battle fractures is another advance of the highest level.

So the contribution of Scots to military medicine continues, and if this account is breathless, it is because the size of the contribution makes it so.

Acknowledgements

I wish to express my great thanks for the very considerable help given me in the preparation of this paper by Major General Robert Scott, MD, FRCS, now Commandant, Royal Army Medical College at Millbank and former Professor of Military Surgery. He kindly gave me access to both original papers and copy material. I should like to thank also Lieutenant Colonel Ian Haywood, the present Professor of Army

Surgery for his help in obtaining papers, and Miss Alison Stevenson, of the Royal College of Surgeons of Edinburgh, who was also very helpful in allowing me access to material.

The Influence of Scotland on North American Medicine

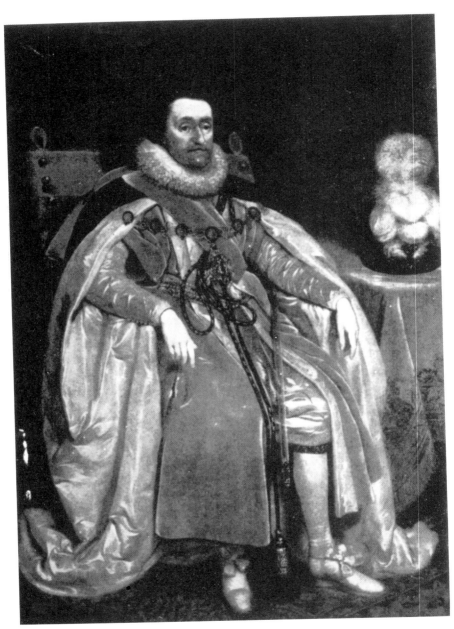

James VI of Scotland and I of England (1566-1625), portrayed by Daniel Mytens in 1621.

Chapter 3

The Influence of Scotland
on North American Medicine

R H Girdwood

The first Scotsman to influence North American medicine in that he influenced, indirectly, much of what developed later there could be said to be King James VI of Scotland and I of England. (Interestingly, had his *Counterblaste to Tobacco*, first written in 1604, been heeded, the present incidence of bronchial carcinoma in the United Kingdom would have been much reduced.)

In 1585 Sir Walter Raleigh, knowing of the discoveries of the Cabots and other explorers and encouraged by Richard Hakluyt in London, settled the first English colony at Roanoke Island, a small piece of land twelve miles long, off the coast of what is now North Carolina. Queen Elizabeth agreed to the name Virginia being given to all the territories in North America to which the English made pretensions at that time. This and other settlements made immediately after it were unsuccessful, but in 1606 James I issued letters patent to a group of London businessmen for the settlement of the Royal colony of Virginia, and in 1607 there arrived in that area three ships under the command of Captain Christopher Newport. There was dissension and disease amongst the colonists and Captain John Smith, the most able of the settlers, assumed control. Medical help was required. In 1624 James I dissolved the Virginia Company because of the chaos reported from there, and in due course the remains of Jamestown, as the main settlement was named, became a part of the town of Williamsburg which had been established close to it.

There were, of course, other English settlements in North America when James died in 1625 and he must in his lifetime have had personal worries because of hostility between his two kingdoms of Scotland and England. He had supported the establishment of a Scottish colony in

33

Nova Scotia under Sir William Alexander in 1621 but although this was a failure it gave Nova Scotia its present name, its flag and its coat of arms. In 1625 Charles I maintained this connection by creating an order of baronets of Nova Scotia, open to Scots, this entitlement being granted at a ceremony on the parade ground of Edinburgh Castle. Strong medical links with the city came only at a much later date.

Those who settled in North America frequently required attention for their illnesses and it was necessary for medical training to be made available. If any settler had some medical experience or knowledge he could pass it on, but this was far from sufficient. James I had a personal interest in the universities of Oxford, Cambridge and Edinburgh, this last being known by his command as King James's College. Oxford and Cambridge could only be entered by students who were members of the Church of England, and neither had a hospital. Edinburgh did not have a medical school. At Aberdeen and St Andrews medical degrees could be purchased, but this was of no practical help and the Glasgow medical school had not yet been established. Padua, Leyden, Utrecht, Montpellier, Paris and Rheims undertook medical training and in the early 18th century a few students from the colonies matriculated at Leyden, but it was not until the Edinburgh Faculty was instituted in 1726 that a solution to the problem became available.

There is no record of the numbers of colonists who came eastwards to Scotland for medical training prior to 1726. Some Scots with a knowledge of medicine went to the New World from a spirit of adventure; others fled their native country because of having supported the defeated Stuart cause.

John Johnston, an Edinburgh apothecary, settled in New York late in the 17th century. Dr Archibald Blair from Aberdeenshire graduated from the University of Edinburgh in 1685 although not in medicine, as the University then offered no such qualification. Nevertheless he appeared in Jamestown about 1690 with practical knowledge of medical matters. However, Jamestown was giving place to Williamsburg, which became the first capital of Virginia, and he moved there to establish a shop, not confining his activities to the sale of medicines or treatment of patients. Of interest is the fact that he is said to have been responsible for the construction of the Raleigh Tavern where the Burgesses in 1774 issued a call for the first Continental Congress which met in Philadelphia on 5 September of that year. Decisions which were taken on that occasion led to the War of Independence.

Before this war, however, there were numerous Scottish doctors in Williamsburg and elsewhere in Virginia. Their names have been listed by various authors and their places of origin are known to have included Aberdeen, Coldstream, Dumfriesshire, Edinburgh, Glasgow, West Lothian and Wigtownshire, i.e. mainly the southern parts of the country. Some sailed at the time when rebel prisoners were being deported to America after the Jacobite rebellions of 1715 and 1745. Unlike the doctors, these were mainly Highland Scots and perhaps about a thousand prisoners in all went to North Carolina, Maryland or Virginia, where they probably received medical attention from Scottish doctors, while American students in Edinburgh must have seen, in the new Royal Infirmary, some of those injured in 1745 or 1746.

In the 17th and 18th centuries most American physicians neither emigrated from Scotland nor went there to be trained. There was a very definite system of apprenticeship, with young medical students between the ages of 14 and 18 entering the office of a local practitioner under a three to seven year indenture. For example, the records show that Michael Wallace, born at Galrigs in Scotland in 1719, was indentured by his uncles to an apprenticeship with Dr Gustavus Brown who had settled in Maryland in 1708. Gustavus Brown himself had studied in Edinburgh, as did a number of his descendants, but this agreement was signed in Glasgow in 1734. Thus Scot could be training Scot in the New World. An alternative was to study with a local practitioner and obtain a certificate of service and proficiency. Many Virginians obtained a basic education at the College of William and Mary in Williamsburg, were apprenticed to a local doctor, and then spent a few years in Edinburgh.

Most of those who crossed the Atlantic to Scotland to study medicine went to Edinburgh rather than elsewhere, but Glasgow graduates in Virginia in the 18th century included Mottrom Ball and William Spence. To confuse matters, it has to be remembered that it was possible to study medicine in one Scottish university but obtain the degree in another one, or to study in Scotland but obtain the degree in Leyden. Mottrom Ball studied in Edinburgh and Glasgow before graduating from the latter in 1790, while Thomas Tarpley studied first in Williamsburg then in Edinburgh but graduated in Leyden in 1773. Blanton stated that 65 colonists from Virginia obtained the Edinburgh MD between 1749 and 1812 while many others obtained training but did not take the degree. Precise numbers are difficult to estimate but Rendall, in a contribution to Anderson and Simpson's volume, calculated that 51 Virginians studied at Edinburgh in the quarter century from 1770 to 1795.

This pattern relates only to Virginia, the source of the majority of American medical students in these early days. The unpopular Union of the Parliaments in 1707 had led to a decline in the status of Edinburgh, prompting the city fathers to make provision for the establishment of an international medical school there. The Deacon of the Incorporation of Surgeon Apothecaries (John Munro), the Lord Provost of Edinburgh (George Drummond) and a group of Fellows of the Royal College of Physicians of Edinburgh had in fact agreed that a university faculty of medicine should be established with a structured medical curriculum, systematic and clinical teaching and an examination that would lead to the granting of a degree. Most of the founders of the medical school were influenced by the teaching they had themselves received at Leyden. Nothing similar was available elsewhere in the British Isles. In 1726 the Faculty of Medicine came into being and in 1729 the small Royal Infirmary was opened. Nine years later William Adam (father of Robert, John and James and hence the progenitor of a most remarkable architectural family) was asked to design a hospital to accommodate 228 patients. Things moved more rapidly than in present times and, despite lack of finance, it was completed by 1748. One wing had already been opened in 1741 and during the Jacobite rising of 1745-6 part of the Royal Infirmary served as a military hospital. It is for this reason that some of the American students may have encountered the results of civil war first in Scotland and later in North America, and it was, of course, possible for Scots' doctors to be involved themselves in both conflicts.

The best known doctor to have such involvement in warfare on both sides of the Atlantic was Hugh Mercer who was born in Aberdeenshire in 1776. He was educated at Marischal College, Aberdeen and, after having obtained a medical training, joined the army of Prince Charles Edward Stuart. After Culloden he had to flee to Philadelphia, and eventually settled in Virginia as a result of an important friendship gained in battle. In 1754 the Virginian militia fought joint forces of French and Indians, after Lt.Col. George Washington had been sent to order the French officer, Col. St Pierre, to surrender Fort Du Quesne, a post at the junction of the Alleghany and Monogahela rivers. The Virginians were unsuccessful, and in 1755 General Braddock was sent from Ireland to march against Fort Du Quesne. Accompanying him in the assault was Hugh Mercer. The attack was a disaster, with heavy casualties on the British side, but amongst the survivors were George Washington and Hugh Mercer.

On 25 November, 1758 Mercer was involved in the successful British attack on Fort Du Quesne, thereafter named Pittsburgh. The friendship which he had formed with George Washington now led him to move to Fredericksburg, reasonably close to Washington's estate at Mount Vernon. He had achieved the rank of Major, but resumed the practice of medicine and opened an apothecary shop. When the Revolution erupted he became a Colonel and was sent to pursue the fourth Earl of Dunmore who was then Governor of Virginia, but was himself seriously injured at the Battle of Princeton. He had been promoted to Brigadier-General, and Washington sent Benjamin Rush to attend to his wounds, but he died on 12 January 1777. Much had happened to him since the Battle of Culloden in 1746, but it is not known whether he still retained a high regard for the unhappy Charles Edward Stuart, now beset by illness, alcoholism and marital problems in his place of exile, the city of Florence.

Another Edinburgh-trained medical man to settle in Fredericksburg was Dr Adam Stephen. He reached America in 1748, but ceased medical practice in 1754 to become a fighting officer under George Washington in both the French and Indian wars and the revolutionary conflict. Stephen rose to the rank of Major-General, but was dismissed for having been intoxicated at the Battle of Germantown on 3 October 1777, despite his brave conduct at the Battle of Brandywine on 11 September of that year. In contrast, William Graham served as a surgeon at the latter battle, and it was after that, in 1783, that he came to Edinburgh to continue his medical studies. Some of the doctors who had trained in Scotland before this war supported the revolutionary cause, others were loyalists and some were neutral. A few were undergoing training in Scotland when the war broke out and remained in order to obtain their medical degrees. Certainly one (Benjamin Waterhouse) was so unhappy in Edinburgh that he completed his studies in Leyden, obtaining an MD degree there in 1780. Dr James Craik from Arbigland near Dumfries studied medicine in Edinburgh. He fought with Washington against the French, then, during the War of Independence, again with Washington's army. Having organised the Medical Department of the forces of Count Rochambeau, he took part in the capitulation ceremony at Yorktown. He then settled in Alexandria, Va., near Mount Vernon. He, with Dr Gustavus Richard

Brown (MD Edin, 1768) and Elisha Cullen Dick (who studied under Benjamin Rush and William Shippen and graduated MD Pennsylvania in 1782), attended Washington in his final illness. Craik had the greatest medical influence over George Washington during a period of many years.

Thomas Jefferson, later active in the struggle for independence, was the prime mover in the formation of a medical school at Williamsburg. Anxious to establish such a school at the William and Mary College, he persuaded James McClurg (MD Edin, 1770) to occupy a chair of medicine from 1779 to 1783. The school did not remain in existence and McClurg became a noted trainer of apprentices in Richmond, Virginia.

In describing Scotland's early influence on North American medicine it has been necessary to devote much of the discussion to a consideration of the Virginians. Such was their numerical supremecy that a Virginia Club was formed in 1761 by the medical students attending Edinburgh University. Attention must now, however, be switched to the Scottish influence on medical affairs elsewhere in North America.

The settlement of Maryland took place in 1633. Gustavus Brown of Dalkeith studied medicine in Edinburgh some time before the establishment of the Faculty of Medicine. While acting as a surgeon's mate he was left behind by his ship in Maryland, a storm having blown up when he was ashore. He remained there and taught his medical skills. He fathered twelve children by his first wife, eight being girls. Of the four sons one — named Richard — survived, but the other three, all given the name Gustavus, died in infancy. He married a second time and had a son and a daughter. The son was Gustavus Richard Brown, to whom reference has already been made. He was the physician who arrived at George Washington's deathbed after he had been vigorously bled by Craik and Dick, possibly for a quinsy.

Gustavus Brown senior's grandson was named Gustavus Brown junior. The son of the Rev. Richard Brown, he was born at Morningside, Edinburgh and qualified in medicine at Edinburgh in 1770. He then settled in Maryland. His brother, William, graduated in medicine in Edinburgh the same year, settled in Alexandria, Va., and on the recommendation of Hugh Mercer succeeded Benjamin Rush as Surgeon General of the Middle Department in the American Army. He wrote a *Pharmacopeia for the Use of Army Hospitals*.

The Scottish influx gained a greater momentum in the second half of the eighteenth century. It is known that about 650 medical students from North America graduated MD in Edinburgh between 1750 and 1850 and that many others took classes without graduating. A much smaller number graduated in Glasgow where there were curricular difficulties. One potential stimulus to this transatlantic interchange was the fact that there were serious problems in Britain about the large numbers of medical graduates being produced by the Scottish universities. Indeed, between 1750 and 1850 just over 500 doctors graduated from English universities (Oxford and Cambridge), but more than 10,000 obtained degrees from Scottish universities. Aberdeen and St Andrews even gave degrees by post, a practice which lowered the standing of all Scottish medical degrees in England; in retaliation the London College of Physicians and later the Society of Apothecaries in London strenuously opposed the recognition of Scottish qualifications. This led many Scottish medical graduates to seek posts overseas, and a significant number went to North America. Scotland also had a considerable impact on the development of North American medical schools, the lead mainly coming from American doctors trained in Edinburgh. It has to be realized, too, that many American doctors, trained in Scotland, subsequently took on medical students as apprentices.

This influence was especially marked in Philadelphia. John Fothergill (1712-80), a Yorkshireman and a Quaker, was an Edinburgh MD of 1736 and a Fellow of the Royal College of Physicians of Edinburgh. He was one Scottish graduate who managed to practise successfully in London and he became noted for his philanthropy. However, his father, a preacher, had visited the American colonies and the son became much interested in medical developments in North America. Benjamin Franklin visited him in 1757, and also visited Edinburgh in 1759. There developed a valuable communication system with Franklin commending the Edinburgh medical school and encouraging American students to visit Fothergill or write to him, and Fothergill sending letters about students both to Franklin and to friends in Edinburgh. William Shippen (MD Edin, 1761), John Morgan (MD Edin, 1763) and Benjamin Rush (MD Edin, 1768) were all influenced by Fothergill, who encouraged the first two to develop a medical school in Philadelphia and in 1762 wrote to James Pemberton in that city suggesting that Morgan and Shippen would be able to develop such a school. In fact Morgan attempted to have the new medical school established under his own control without Shippen and, although they continued to quarrel, the Philadelphia medical school was founded in 1765, based on the Edinburgh model. Adam Kuhn, also an Edinburgh graduate, joined them in 1768, and the following year Benjamin Rush, later to become famous as the only medical signatory of the Declaration of Independence, joined them as Professor of Chemistry.

Rush had arrived at Liverpool on 22 October 1766 and had written immediately to Benjamin Franklin asking him to approach his friends in Edinburgh on behalf of Rush and a fellow student, Jonathan Potts. Potts left Edinburgh abruptly the following year because his fiancée was grieving for him, and graduated MD in Philadelphia in 1771. Benjamin Rush had a letter of introduction to the influential Sir Alexander Dick and for the rest of his life was most appreciative of his student days in Scotland, being particularly impressed by the teaching of Cullen. In one of his letters he says 'My halcyon days have been spent in Edinburgh'. Despite this, Rush believed the signs augured well for a medical school in Philadelphia, and on 20 January 1768 he wrote that 'Boarding is now become so excessive high in Edinburgh that few students will be able to come hereafter from America'.

The College of Physicians of Philadelphia was founded in 1787, and of the initial twenty-four Fellows, there were eight Edinburgh graduates. In the same city the American Medical Society was a student society based on that of the Edinburgh students, the Royal Medical Society. Casper Wistar (MD Edin, 1786), after whom the plant wisteria is named, came from Philadelphia and was a student President of the Royal Medical Society, one of eight American students to be so honoured.

Scottish graduates were also active in other areas of North America. In Philadelphia there was a suitable hospital for clinical instruction, but not so in New York. John Jay (MD Edin, 1763) had proposed a medical school, but in 1767 the trustees of King's College invited six physicians and surgeons in New York to found a Medical Faculty. The impetus now came largely from Samuel Bard (MD Edin, 1765) who became Professor of the Theory and Practice of Physic, having been supported in the project by his father, John Bard (1716-99), a well esteemed New York surgeon.

King's College was disrupted by war and closed down, but in 1787 the Medical Faculty of what was now Columbia College was opened. There were five professors and these included Samuel Bard, Samuel Mitchell (MD Edin, 1786) and Nicholas Romayne (MD Edin, 1779). The last of these broke away to found a rival medical school. One of his pupils, David Hosack (1769-1835), a medical graduate of Philadelphia, who had also studied in Edinburgh, attempted to found his own medical school in 1826. Such private medical schools did not survive, but Hosack, whose father came from Elgin in Scotland, established the Elgin Botanic Garden on a site now occupied by the Rockefeller Centre. A plaque there commemorates his name.

The doctors in the Carolinas in the 18th century were largely trained in Scotland. They included John Moultrie, Lionel Chalmers, Tucker Harris and Alexander Garden. Gardenias are named after the last-named, and the word poinsettia commemorates the name of Dr JR Poinset who studied medicine in Edinburgh early in the 19th century. Elsewhere on the eastern seaboard, Nathan Smith, a Harvard graduate, desired to study medicine and did so in Edinburgh at the end of the 18th century. He established a school of medicine at Dartmouth College in New Hampshire and later was Professor of Surgery at Yale.

An equally strong Scottish influence can be traced in development further north, in Canada. James McGill emigrated to Montreal from Glasgow and died in 1813. He left part of his estate for the foundation of a university with a medical school. The medical officers of the Montreal General Hospital were anxious for this to be done and, with the support of Lord Dalhousie, there was established, in November 1824, a medical school with twenty-five students, the name adopted by it at this time being the Montreal Medical Institution. Those involved at this stage were Andrew Holmes (MD Edin, 1819; chemistry, pharmacy, botany), John Stephenson (MD Edin, 1820; anatomy, physiology, surgery), William Robertson (studied at Edinburgh; midwifery) and William Caldwell (studied at Edinburgh; practice of physic). This Institution was later constituted as the Medical Faculty of McGill University and, in 1832, it received a Royal Charter. In the same year Thomas Fargues (MD Edin, 1811) was appointed Professor of Medicine.

Quite apart from this early and profound Edinburgh influence, the links were maintained and, in 1899, a new teaching hospital based on the architectural plans of Edinburgh Royal Infirmary was opened on the slopes of Mount Royal.

L'Université de Montréal was formed in 1920 by the union of L'Ecole de Médecine et Chirurgie de Montréal, the first French medical school in Montreal and L'Université de Laval de Montréal. The first of these French medical schools was founded in 1843 by a group of five doctors which included three Edinburgh graduates. These were Dr Francis Arnoldi (MD Edin, 1823) first President of the School, Francis Badgley (MD Edin, 1829) and William McNider (MD Edin, 1836).

There was some Edinburgh influence at the time of the foundation of the medical schools in Quebec, Toronto, Queen's College, (Kingston, Ontario) and Dalhousie University, Halifax, Nova Scotia. The Halifax initiative deserves a special mention. Of the fourteen doctors practising in 1845, all but one had studied at Edinburgh. A driving force behind the establishment of a Medical Faculty was Dr Charles Tupper (1821-1915; MD Edin, 1843). He played an important role in the Canadian Union of 1864 which led to the formation of the Dominion. Sir Charles Tupper was Prime Minister of Canada in 1896.

When I was a medical student there were several Canadian undergraduates studying medicine at Edinburgh, but now the policy, in the light of the number of applicants, is not to take undergraduate medical students from countries which have their own medical schools. However, each university in the United Kingdom has its own policy. At the present time the North American students usually attend North American universities, but at the postgraduate level there is still an exchange of teachers and of students. The graduate in medicine is fortunate in that no matter where he travels he will be able to make friends with colleagues and enrich his experience and knowledge. It is a source of particular pride to we Scots that our predecessors, in North America and elsewhere, have done so much to encourage such relations.

CHAPTER 4

Scottish Man–Midwives in 18th Century London

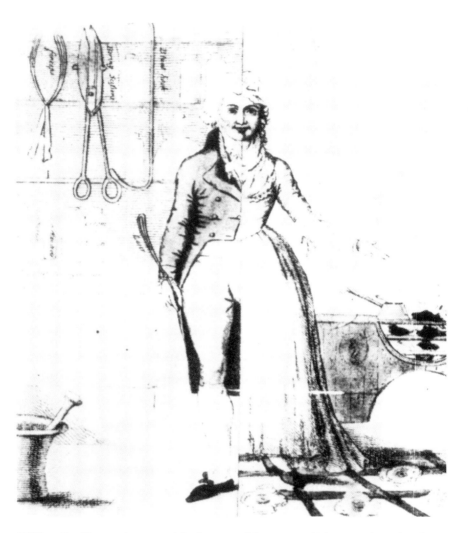

William Smellie was almost certainly the target of the cartoon which appeared in John Blunt's "Man Midwifery Dissected" in 1793 – three decades after Smellie's death.

Chapter 4
Scottish Man-Midwives in 18th Century London
J Willocks

In the second half of the 17th century, the art of midwifery in Britain appeared to be in an unsatisfactory state.[1] Most of its practitioners were uneducated women of the type that Dickens later caricatured in Sarah Gamp. Men did not take up the practice of midwifery merely to help suffering humanity. The Chamberlens invented the forceps and managed to keep it as a family secret for about 200 years to their own great profit. It was knowledge of the forceps that gave men the 'key to the lying-in room', and introduced the man-midwife into obstetric practice in this country.[2] Despite much opposition obstetrics became a respectable profession in the first half of the 18th century and three of its leading practitioners were knighted — Sir David Hamilton by Queen Anne, Sir Richard Manningham by George I and Sir Fielding Ould by George II. Of this last knighthood a wit wrote:

'Sir Fielding Ould is made a knight
He should have been a Lord by right
For then each lady's prayer would be
Oh Lord! Good Lord deliver me'.[3]

Scotsmen played an important part in the development of obstetrics in the 18th century and the three greatest of them practised in London — William Smellie, James Douglas and William Hunter.

William Smellie
William Smellie was born at Lanark in 1697[4] and being 'very idle and dull at school was taken more up with carving and painting than his books'. He obtained his medical education as apprentice to Dr John Gordon in Glasgow where Tobias Smollett, Smellie's lifelong friend, was probably a student. Smellie started practice in Lanark in 1720, but

45

no formal medical qualifications were conferred on him until 1733, when he was admitted as a fellow of what is now The Royal College of Physicians and Surgeons of Glasgow. In 1745 the University of Glasgow conferred on him the degree of MD.

For nineteen years he was a general practitioner in the arduous conditions of rural Lanarkshire and during that time established such a reputation in midwifery that he was called into consultation in various parts of the country. Obstructed labour was common and the loss of the child a frequent occurrence. Smellie was dissatisfied with his results and went to study in London. He was already 42 years of age but his years of achievement were still to come. He went to learn and stayed to teach, not returning to Lanark till he retired twenty years later.[5]

His own words describe this remarkable change in his life:

'During the first year of my practice, when I was called to lingering cases, which were often occasioned by the imprudent methods used by unskilful midwives to hasten labour, I have been told that the patient had been in severe labour for many hours, and sometimes days, and that now I was called to prevent her from dying with the child in her belly. Thus solicited, if the head was at the upper part of the pelvis, I commonly turned the child and brought it by the feet; and thus, if small, it was usually saved, provided it was not dead before my arrival; but when the head was large, or the pelvis narrow and distorted, the force necessary to extract it was often the occasion of its death.

On the other hand, when the head was so low in the pelvis that I could not raise it in the uterus in order to be turned, I was obliged to perforate the cranium with the scissors and extract with my fingers, assisted by the blunt hook.

In order to avoid this loss of children, which gave me great uneasiness, I procured a pair of French forceps — but found them so long and so ill contrived, that they by no means answered the purposes for which they were intended. I afterwards perused the treatises of Chapman and Giffard, who had frequently saved children by a contrivance of this kind; and actually made a journey to London in order to acquire further information on this subject. Here I saw nothing was to be learned; and by the advice of the late ingenious Dr Stewart, who was my particular friend, I proceeded to Paris where courses on midwifery at that time were given by Gregoire. There likewise I was much disappointed in my expectation ... as for the forceps, he taught his pupils to introduce them at random, and pull with great force . . . Little satisfied with his manner of instructing, I considered that there was a possibility of forming machines, which should so exactly imitate real women and children, as to exhibit to the learner all the difficulties that happen in midwifery and such I actually contrived and made by dint of uncommon labour and application ... In a word, I diligently attended to the course and operations of nature which occurred in my practice, regulating and improving myself by that infallible standard; nor did I reject the hints of other writers and practitioners, from whose suggestions, I own, I have derived much useful instruction'.[6]

Smellie started to practise and teach midwifery in London on his return from Paris. He lived and worked in Soho. He offered to attend, gratis, poor women at their confinements in their own houses, provided that his students were allowed to accompany him. As there were no maternity hospitals when he started practice in London, this was an offer of considerable value. Each pupil, in addition to his fee for the course, contributed a sum into a common fund for the patients. During ten years he gave 280 courses in midwifery to more than 900 pupils and in that series over 1,100 poor women were delivered.[7]

Smellie carried on his teaching practice against a veritable blizzard of opposition which pursued him even beyond the grave for he appears as one of the villains in an early Victorian book entitled *Man Midwifery Exposed*.[8] Some of Smellie's opponents were beneath contempt, but the most formidable of them is certainly worth a mention. She was Mrs Elizabeth Nihell, who was one of the most famous midwives of the period.[9] She was well aware that man-midwives were gaining popularity and female midwives were losing it entirely because of the obstetric forceps. The summary of her argument was that instruments, meaning forceps, were never necessary, therefore man-midwives were never necessary. Her treatise on the art of midwifery, published in 1760, was dedicated 'to all fathers, mothers and likely soon to be either'. She soon diverted from the interests of these prospective parents to lash out at man-midwives. 'That multitude of disciples of Dr Smellie, trained up at the feet of his artificial doll, or, in short, those self constituted man-midwives made out of broken barbers, tailors, even pork butchers, for I know myself one of this last trade, who after passing half his life in stuffing sausages, is turned an intrepid physician and man-midwife'. Later she became more personal and referred, vividly if incoherently, to the master himself. 'The delicate fist of a great horse-godmother of a he-midwife, however softened his figure might be by his pocket nightgown being of flowered calico or his cap of office tied with pink and silver ribbon'. Mrs Nihell recognised Smellie as the great leader of a new movement towards man-midwifery which she saw might take both money and reputation away from women. Man-midwives she said, were a band of mercenaries who palmed themselves off upon pregnant women under cover of their 'crotchets, knives, scissors, spoons, pinchers, fillets and speculums, all of which, and especially their forceps, whether Flemish, Dutch, Irish, French or English, bare or covered, long or short, straight or crooked, windowed or not windowed, are totally useless or rather worse than good for nothing, being never but dangerous and often destructive'. This extended dispute gave midwifery a news value which it had never had before and produced public interest which stimulated the development of maternity hospitals in Britain.

William Smellie himself preserved a dignified silence in this controversy and, in contrast to the scurrility of his opponents, his concept of the qualities required for the practice of midwifery was of the most elevated kind:

'Those who intend to practice midwifery, ought first of all to make themselves masters of anatomy, and acquire a competent knowledge of surgery and physic; because of their connection with the obstetric art. He ought to take the best opportunities he can find of being well instructed; and of practising under a Master, before he attempts to deliver by himself . . .

But, over and above the advantage of a good education, he ought to be endowed with a natural sagacity, resolution and prudence, together with that humanity which adorns the owner, and never fails of being agreeable to the distressed patient; in consequence of this virtue, he will assist the poor as well as the rich, behaving always with charity and compassion. He ought to act and speak with the utmost delicacy of decorum, and never violate the trust reposed in him, so as to harbour the least immoral or indecent design; but demean himself in all respects suitable to the dignity of his profession'.[10]

Smellie's teaching is contained in his three-volume *Treatise on the Theory and Practice of Midwifery*. The first of these is concerned with systematic teaching while the second and third contain details of 531 illustrative cases from the author's experience. This work was published between 1751 and 1764, the last volume appearing after Smellie's death. In the preparation of the treatise he was assisted by his friend, Smollett.

Smellie's description of normal labour is one of his great contributions to obstetrics. He showed that the fetal head usually engaged in the pelvic brim with the forehead to one side and the occiput to the other:

'Thus the widest part of the head is turned to the widest part of the pelvis, and the narrow part of the head from ear to ear, applied to the narrow part of the pelvis between the pubes and the sacrum'.

In the lower part of the pelvis, Smellie pointed out, the head rotates so that the occiput comes under the pubic arch and:

'The forehead then turns into the hollow at the lower end of the sacrum, and now again the narrow part of the head is turned to the narrow part of the pelvis'.

This was the first clear and coherent description in the whole history of midwifery of the movements of the head in relation to the pelvis during birth, controverting all the theory and superstitution of the past and based solely on Smellie's own clinical observations and independent reasoning.[11] Such an observation may seem commonplace today, but it was revolutionary when first penned by Smellie.

Smellie insisted on the importance of pelvic measurement and was the first to measure the diagonal conjugate. This was the most important contribution ever made to clinical pelvimetry. He also described the various types of contracted pelvis and the mechanism of labour in these cases, giving a brilliant account of the aetiology of the flat pelvis caused by rickets. His demonstration of the scientific and rational use of the forceps made operative obstetrics humane. The barbarities previously practised had 'produced a general clamour among the women, who observed that when recourse was had to the assistance of a man-midwife, either the mother or child, or both, were lost'.

Despite Smellie's advocacy of the forceps, his methods were conservative: 'In my practice,' he wrote, 'I have very seldom occasion for the assistance of that or any other instrument'. He went on to advise young practitioners 'above all things, to beware of being too hasty in offering assistance while Nature is of herself able to effectuate the delivery'.

The luminous clarity of Smellie's case records cannot be bettered in medical literature. His simple, vivid language gives the reader — even 200 years later — a sense of participation in the cases and is in salutary contrast to the dull impersonality, the muddled jargon and pseudo-Graeco-Roman verbosity of much modern medical writing.

Smellie was a talented painter in oils and could be a painter in words too. The following extract gives some flavour of his style:

'In the year 1751 I was called to Fenchurch Street by one of my pupils, who with an old midwife, was attending a patient pretty much advanced in years, in labour of a first child. Everything was in a right way for safe delivery; but as the case was tedious and lingering both the woman and her friends were impatient and had sent for an old blundering pretender in the neighbourhood, who told the patient that she was in the utmost danger if she was not immediately delivered. He said he hoped he would save her life, but the child was dead already; and he called in another midwife who confirmed what he asserted.

The woman's pains had been vigorous, but these dismal operations frightened her so much that when I arrived they were quite gone off. After conversing with the patient we (all five) went to another room when the parties began to quarrel: I called the old blustering practitioner aside and told him my opinion that the woman was in no danger, but by time and patience I hoped would be safely delivered. Nay, I threatened to have him called before the College if he insisted on any violent operation; then he quitted the house with his associate. After his departure we had time to soothe and encourage the woman. As she had got little sleep we gave her a draught with 30 drops of Tinct. Thebaic and the midwife delivered her safely next day'.[12]

In 1754 Smellie published his *Anatomical Tables*[13] to illustrate his *Treatise*, with pictures by Jan van Rymsdyk, Peter Camper and some by Smellie himself. Van Rymsdyk's original drawings were bought by William Hunter and are now in Glasgow University Library.

In 1759 he retired from London to Lanark where he built a small country house. Here he lived quietly, revising his final volume of cases until his death on 5 March 1763 at the age of 66. Though happily married for thirty-nine years he had no children. 'When not engaged in business', he wrote, 'his greatest pleasure was home' and his retirement was enlivened by reading, painting and music, to all of which he was devoted. When he died he left his library and collection of musical instruments to the school at Lanark and the books may now be seen in the Lindsay Institute there.

Smellie's work is of value for all time and his position as 'the master of British midwifery' is assured. As S J Cameron wrote in 1957, 'The edifice of reason which he erected has lasted for two centuries and will do so forever'.

James Douglas

Compared with Smellie, James Douglas seems a shadowy figure, despite the fact that every medical student knows his name from 'the pouch of Douglas' or, as the Continentals say, 'the Douglas'[14]. There is no portrait of him and only one description of him as 'a fair faced, long nosed gentleman'. The preservation of his memory is largely due to his great pupil, William Hunter, who inherited all his papers and kept them carefully.[15] From the study of these archives, Douglas emerges as a great scholar and scientist and a prominent medical man in the social scene of 18th century London.[16]

James Douglas was born in 1675 at Badds, West Calder, near Edinburgh, into a prosperous land owning family. He may have studied arts at Edinburgh University and certainly his notebook, compiled at the age of 19, shows him as a sophisticated, shrewd and witty youth, reflecting on life in aphorisms and verses in the manner of the time. He seems later to have studied in Holland and assembled a medical library in Utrecht in 1698. The library included eighty medical books and some of general interest including *Don Quixote* in French (this was the book which Sydenham suggested 'was better than any medical text books'). He took his medical degree at Rheims in July 1699 and started practice in London in 1700. Records exist of over 200 cases between 1700 and 1712. These suggest that he was closely associated with Paul Chamberlen of the obstetric forceps family and that he acted as a locum for him. His patients were mainly working class people and he recorded their clinical histories with care. One Mrs Dawson, after a dose of medicine that worked 'four times upwards and seven or eight times downwards', was next day described as 'lightsomer'. Another, Mrs Bruce, left him 'for a quack who promised to make her as well as ever in less than 2 months' but she died in less than that time. He recorded one unfortunate attempt at forceps delivery, when 'I was sent for by Mrs Agnew the midwife to lay a poor woman'. He applied the forceps 'but could never fasten the thing so as to be able to pull by reason they were not made right'. After trying for more than an hour he had to give up, whereupon 'I went for young Dr Hugh Chamberlen but he excused himself from coming . . . Dr Johnson was sent for, he lessened the head so brought it away' — in other words the patient was delivered by craniotomy.

There are no detailed case histories after the year 1712 but it appears that, while continuing to treat the poor he began at this time to acquire a fashionable practice among the aristocracy. From the start of his time in London, Douglas also studied anatomy — both human and comparative — and numerous notes of his dissections survive. In 1706 he began to lecture on anatomy, giving a course which, for the first time in England, taught comparative anatomy and demonstrated microscopic details. On Wednesday 4 December 1706 he was admitted a Fellow of the Royal Society by the President, Sir Isaac Newton.

In 1720 James Douglas became an Honorary Fellow of the Royal College of Physicians (a rare distinction for one who was not a graduate of Oxford or Cambridge) and soon after this became known at Court. In 1725 he obtained a grant of £500 from King George I to enable him 'to communicate the observations and discoveries he has made in anatomy, both human and comparative and in the diseases incident to women'. The King may have become interested in Douglas's work through one of the Court physicians. He certainly did not require his services as an obstetrician, for he had left his wife shut up in Hanover and his mistresses at the English Court were past the age of child bearing.

Douglas studied the reproductive system in the non-pregnant woman and at various stages in pregnancy. He was the first to describe the structure of the round ligaments of the uterus and he made interesting observations on the placenta. There is no doubt that the illustrations which he made on the pregnant uterus were the inspiration for William Hunter's great anatomical masterpiece.[17]

In 1730 he published his famous treatise, *A Description of the Peritoneum*. This was his most important anatomical work and it is in this book and in these words that Douglas described the pouch named after him. 'Where the peritoneum leaves the foreside of the rectum it makes an angle and changes its course upwards and forwards over the bladder'.[18] Douglas's interest in the peritoneum is further shown by his drawings, hitherto unpublished, showing inversion of the uterus, one of the most dramatic complications of obstetrics. By the time Douglas was called to attend the patient it was too late to save her life but at least he had the interest of preparing a fine dissection.[19]

James Douglas intended to publish a clinical book called *An Introduction to the Knowledge and Cure of Disease Incident to Women and the Improvement of the Practice of Midwifery* but like many of his other schemes it never reached the press. He was, however, involved in the greatest obstetric sensation of the 18th century, the case of Mary Toft.[20] Mary Toft was the wife of a poor journeyman clothier of Godalming in Surrey who, in the first week of November 1726, gave birth to a rabbit. Further rabbits followed and Mary became the talk of the town. Medical opinion was fascinated but not entirely sceptical. It was a credulous age as is our own. For a woman to give birth to rabbits might be rare, but not inherently improbable. John Howard, a respectable man-midwife of Guildford, delivered many of these rabbits which had been observed to leap about inside the uterus for hours before delivery. In the case of the bigger and better rabbits, this movement might last for as long as thirty hours. 'This particular fact was unanimously agreed on by most of the people of Guildford'. Mary was such a medical miracle that Mr Howard suggested that both patient and obstetrician should receive a government pension. However, the government decided sensibly that the case should be the subject of an enquiry by the two most eminent obstetricians of the day, Sir Richard Manningham and Dr James Douglas. In their presence she confessed that the rabbits had been introduced into her vagina by a woman accomplice 'who told her that she had now no occasion to work for her living as formerly for she would put her in a way of getting a very good livelihood and promised continually to supply her with rabbits, and she should therefore accept part of the gain'. This notorious case probably increased the reputation of James Douglas, for in 1727 he was appointed physician to Queen Caroline, wife of the recently crowned King George II. Caroline's political influence was enormous and Prime Minister Robert Walpole owed much of his power to her consistent support. Douglas was now in the corridors of power and the Royal Family must have thought highly of him for when their daughter Ann, Princess of Orange, was in 1734 thought to be pregnant, Douglas was sent over to Holland to look after her. For this service the King awarded him an annuity of £500.

James Douglas continued to work on his various research projects, including his osteology[21] which, had it been completed, might have been the greatest anatomical work of the 18th century. Whether because of the multiplicity of his interests, lack of organisation or the demands of a busy practice, most of his research never reached publication. Douglas had a number of assistants working with him including his brother George, who became the fourth brother of the family to be elected a Fellow of the Royal Society. Another assistant whom Douglas supported in his election to the Royal Society was James Parsons, who used his artistic talent to make many anatomical and zoological drawings. Douglas was always generous to poor people who had fallen on bad times and one of those whom he employed was Samuel Boyes, an Irish graduate of Glasgow University and a poet. Boyes was too poor to buy a second shirt so invented paper collars and cuffs to supply its place when his one shirt was washed. Douglas's interests extended beyond science into language and literature. He wrote on English, French, Latin and Greek grammar and on English pronunciation. His major literary interest was the poems of Horace. This may have been responsible for his acquaintance with Alexander Pope who greatly admired and imitated the Roman poet. Pope referred to Douglas as: 'a physician of great learning and no less taste, above all curious in what related to Horace of whom he collected every edition, translation and comment'. Pope mentioned Douglas in the *Dunciad* published in 1727, in the often quoted couplet:

'There all the learned shall at the labour stand
and Douglas lend his soft obstetric hand'[22]

Also through his interest in Horace, Douglas came into contact with the brothers Robert and Andrew Foulis of Glasgow who produced beautiful editions of the Greek and Latin Classics. When William Hunter arrived in London he carried with him an introduction from the Foulis brothers to James Douglas, who at that time was looking for a new assistant because Parsons had recently left. William Hunter left Smellie in the autumn of 1741 to become assistant to Douglas and tutor to his son, who was studying medicine.

Douglas had married as his second wife Martha Wilkes (aunt to the notorious John Wilkes) and there were two surviving children — Martha Jane born in 1716 and William George born in 1725. It is believed that William Hunter became engaged to Martha Jane Douglas but she died while Hunter and William George were in Paris attending anatomy lectures in 1744.

In fact, the happy relationship between James Douglas and William Hunter had lasted less than a year for Douglas died in 1742. William Hunter described the scene in a letter to his mother: 'I went in, he snatched my hand and spoke a few words. Immediately his fancy wandered and though he could not talk sensibly, yet he still knew me and would not let me go out of the room. I sat on his bed till afternoon, when he expired with his hand locked in mine'.[23] This, however, did not end Hunter's association with the Douglas family for he lived on with them until 1749, being joined in the household in 1742 by his brother James who stayed for a year, and then by John in 1748. Young William George Douglas did not live up to expectations. He was a complete spendthirft and although Hunter lent him considerable sums of money he had eventually to abandon him.[24]

Despite their brief association together, the influence of James Douglas on William Hunter was immense. Not only did he start Hunter's medical career by commencing him as a pupil in surgery in St George's Hospital but he provided the inspiration for almost all of his later research work. Douglas's collection of anatomical specimens, described as 'the best collection that either is or ever was in the possession of any single man', may have been the basis of William Hunter's great collection.

At the age of 19 James Douglas wrote in his notebook, 'Fame is got by indefatigable labour'. This could have served as a motto for William Hunter also.

William Hunter

William Hunter arrived in London in the summer of 1741 aged 23, with some introductions in his pocket and nothing to declare but his genius. He had been a student in the Arts Faculty of Glasgow University for five years, a medical apprentice with Dr William Cullen in Hamilton, and had attended lectures by Monro and others in Edinburgh University. When he arrived in London he lodged for some months as a pupil with William Smellie before joining the Douglas household. Smellie's teaching influenced him greatly. Hunter was fortunate to have his initial training in midwifery from such a master and in later years he referred to Smellie frequently in his lectures.[25]

Hunter's career developed in rather a different manner from that of Smellie. William Smellie, despite his great reputation, was said to be personally large and clumsy and rather awkward and unpleasing in manner, 'so that he never rose into great estimation among persons of rank'. William Hunter rose to the top. His elevation was initially due to James Douglas who introduced him to his aristocratic midwifery practice. Throughout his career Smellie was dealing with difficult cases among the London poor and was frequently involved in emergency situations — the type of practice that has been called 'fire brigade obstetrics'. By contrast, Hunter's practice dealt with more normal cases among the upper classes and this strengthened his natural conservatism.

Hunter was the ideal obstetric consultant. His appearance was dapper and elegant and his manner was attractive and gentlemanly. In his teaching he stressed the social qualities as well as the technical skills of the man-midwife. 'It is not mere safe delivery of the woman will recommend an accoucheur, but a sagacious well conducted behaviour of tenderness, assiduity and delicacy'. This civilised, sophisticated attitude certainly helped his practice.

In 1748 Hunter was appointed to the staff of the Middlesex Hospital which was the first general hospital in Britain to have a maternity department[26] and in 1749 he was appointed to the staff of the British Lying-In Hospital, which was the precursor of Queen Charlotte's. At this stage in his career Hunter's practice was favoured by fortune, for the two most fashionable London consultants disappeared from the scene — Sir Richard Manningham died and Dr Sandys retired. Aristocratic patients then flocked to Hunter and he gained the favour of the Prime Minister, John Stuart, third Earl of Bute. Lord Bute negotiated the marriage of George III with Princess Sophia Charlotte of Mecklenburg-Strelitz, an unknown girl of 17 from a minor German court. Charlotte had an arduous journey to London. She arrived at St

James's Palace at three o'clock in the afternoon of 8 September 1761, after having travelled with scarcely a break for three weeks. The wedding took place six hours later at 9 pm. Supper followed at 11 pm, and the Royal pair retired to bed about 2 am — scarcely a promising start to married life. Yet the King and Queen were idyllically happy for many years. Charlotte of course had not come to be happy, but to bear an heir to the throne and ensure the Royal succession. In this she was overwhelmingly successful.[27] She lost no time in becoming pregnant. The medical and nursing attendants on Queen Charlotte during her first pregnancy and labour were the Royal surgeon, Mr Caesar Hawkins, the Royal accoucheur, Dr William Hunter and the Royal midwife, Mrs Draper. Hunter recorded the events of Queen Charlotte's first three confinements in a small leather bound notebook, now in Glasgow University Library.[28] Prince George (later George IV) was born in August 1762, Prince Frederick (later 'the Grand Old Duke of York') in August 1763 and Prince William (later William IV) in August 1765. Mrs Draper appeared to be in supreme command on these occasions but after that she disappeared from the scene. Dr Hunter then came into his own. The King and Queen trusted him and treated him as a personal friend. Queen Charlotte had fifteen children, thirteen of whom survived into adult life. It could be said that Dr Hunter during his long career as Royal accoucheur behaved rather like the House of Lords in the Napoleonic Wars and 'did nothing in particular and did it very well'.[29] He certainly practised what he preached and allowed nature to take its course.

Hunter gloried in his obstetric conservatism and probably exaggerated it in his lectures. 'We are greatly improved in midwifery within these 20 years past. What is the great improvement? Why, I am proud to have a share in it. It is bringing it back to nature'.[30] His practical and humane attitude comes down to us in the notes of his lectures taken verbatim by some of his students. He lectured on gynaecological subjects, including abnormal menstruation, dysmenorrhea, dyspareunia, the menopause, leucorrhoea, cancer of the uterus and prolapse, and on obstetric subjects including childbed fever (which baffled him) and haemorrhage and eclampsia (which scared him). 'There are two things at the time of labour which I am frightened at (all the others I don't care a sixpence for) — one is a Flooding and the other Convulsions'. He taught gentleness in operative obstetrics:

'Whatever operation we perform in midwifery, as introducing the hand to examine, must be done with a degree of firmness but so gradually as if the woman was asleep and we meant to do it without waking her . . . Never wish, gentlemen, to gain reputation by doing business quick; always take time, particularly in applying the forceps. When the pain is off unlock them that you may not squeeze the child's head. When the head is delivered I often take away the forceps that I may have my hand more at liberty to support the woman. In a few cases I think the forceps a useful instrument. To a poor woman that is quite exhausted they may be of considerable service, but I wish to God they had never been contrived. I am convinced the forceps has killed three, I may say ten women to one that it has saved, and therefore we should never use it on any occasion but where it is absolutely necessary'.[30]

There is no doubt that as a lecturer William Hunter was brilliant, and his performance rivalled that of the great actor David Garrick. (Incidentally, Hunter took care not to lecture when Garrick was performing at the nearby Haymarket Theatre). Hunter was a master of the telling phrase and vivid anecdote drawn from his own experience. 'When I can be of any service telling a failure of my own, I shall relate it readily, though not with that pleasure as a case wherein I have been successful'. The lectures were delivered in a style which even the most distinguished of his listeners, who included Adam Smith, Edmund Burke and Edward Gibbon, would have been proud to emulate. Hunter presented anatomy in a way that could be appreciated not only by members of his own profession, but by men of culture from other walks of life.

William Hunter had no doubt about the vital importance of anatomy in medical education. 'Anatomy is', he wrote, 'the only solid foundation of medicine; it is to the physician and surgeon what geometry is to the astronomer. It discovers and ascertains truth, overturns superstition and vulgar error, and checks the enthusiasm of theorists and sects in medicine, to whom perhaps more of the human species has fallen sacrifice than to the sword itself or to pestilence'.[31]

One of the great objects of William Hunter's life was to set up a school of scientific medicine in London. To promote this, he addressed a memorial in 1765 to Mr Grenville, the Prime Minister, asking for a grant of a piece of ground upon which Hunter himself proposed to spend six or seven thousand pounds in erecting a suitable building. Hunter also offered to endow a professorship in perpetuity. The government refused his offer.

William Hunter eventually decided to go ahead with his plan at his own expense. In 1766, he bought a large house at No 16 Great Windmill Street and asked Robert Mylne, the Scottish architect of Blackfriars Bridge, to rebuild it for him, providing him with a residence, museum, library, anatomical theatre and dissecting rooms.

Hunter moved there from Jermyn Street in 1768 and it was his home for the rest of his life.

William Hunter's research work, like that of his master James Douglas, covered the whole field of anatomy. For example, he made important discoveries about arterio-venous aneurysm, congenital heart disease, congenital hernia, the lachrymal ducts, the seminiferous tubules in the testicle and the lymphatic system. His great masterpiece was *The Anatomy of the Human Gravid Uterus*.[32] This was a subject which had attracted his attention since the early days when he had worked with William Smellie and James Douglas. He was fascinated by the way the child developed and the way that the uterus became adapted to receive and nourish it. In 1750, he had his first opportunity to examine a complete specimen. 'A woman died suddenly when very near the end of her pregnancy; the body was procured before any sensible putrefaction had begun; the season of the year was favourable to dissection; the injection of the blood vessels proved successful'. Having secured the specimen and made the dissection, he employed the best artist he could find to present it in graphic form. This artist was Jan van Rymsdyk, whose drawings, made in red chalk, are of great delicacy. Hunter directed Rymsdyk to make his pictures an accurate representation of what was actually seen. 'Every part was represented as it was found: not so much as one joint of a finger having been moved to show any part more distinctly, or to give more picturesque effect'. For the material to be prepared in book form, Hunter required an engraver and a printer. He was fortunate in the choice of both. Sir Robert Strange, the greatest engraver of his time, was a personal friend and gave his services free. To print the great work, Hunter commissioned John Baskerville of Birmingham, whose fine editions of the Greek and Latin classics were well known to him.

It took twenty-four years to complete. The finished result was a scientific and artistic triumph. In his preface to the book, Hunter acknowledged the assistance of Strange and Baskerville and gave a generous tribute to his brother John but made no mention of Rymsdyk, although his masterly drawings, made over many years, contributed so much to the book's success.[33] William Hunter finished his lecture course of 1775 by demonstrating to the class the plates from the *Gravid Uterus* and stated 'these plates were made from drawings that were taken by Mr Rymsdyk from twelve different subjects, so that they are all exactly after nature'. He concluded, 'I have now finished twenty years of lectures. However, as I presume I am still approved of, I propose twenty years more to begin next October, and after this is over, I propose to settle in the world and to take to me a wife'.[34]

The scientific value of *The Anatomy of the Gravid Uterus* lies in its marvellous description of fetal development from the earliest stages and in the original observations which Hunter made regarding the decidua and the maternal and fetal circulations. These subjects are described in detail in Hunter's manuscript *Description of the Pregnant Uterus*, which was left unpublished at the time of his death.

The Anatomical Collection at Glasgow University preserves Hunter's specimens of the human ovum from the earliest stages, showing the changes in the villi of the chorion, the formation of the placenta, arrangement of the decidua and development and growth of the embryo from about the third week after conception.[35]

Hunter demonstrated clearly the separation between the maternal and fetal circulations. This was probably his most important observation. He wrote, 'It seems incontestable that the human placenta, like that of the quadruped, is composed of two distinct parts, though blended together, viz. an umbilical, which may be considered as part of the fetus, and an uterine, which belongs to the mother; that each of these parts has its peculiar system of arteries and veins, and its peculiar circulation'.[36] Hunter goes on to say that the first time he demonstrated this was in the year 1743. Unfortunately this great discovery was the cause of a serious quarrel with his brother John. Time has substantiated William's views on the structure of the placenta, and the priority of his discovery.

The Anatomy of the Human Gravid Uterus is one of the greatest works of medical illustration ever published, its only rival in artistic merit being the *De Human Corporis Fabrica* of Vesalius. The significance of the discoveries it embodies about the placental circulation and the nature of the decidua are as important to fetal physiology as the work of Harvey on the circulation of the blood is to the adult.

The title page of Hunter's *Gravid Uterus* bears the proud inscription that he was Professor of Anatomy to the Royal Academy. This was an appointment which gave him particular pleasure. The Royal Academy of Art had been established by King George III in 1768 and thereafter Hunter gave lectures and demonstrations on the structure of the human body, particularly the muscles.[37] Through his connection with the Royal Family and his widespread social and political contacts[38], William Hunter had a place in what was intellectually by far the best society of the kingdom, a society in which no talent or accomplishment was wanting, and in which the art of conversation was cultivated with splendid success. Alexander Carlyle[39] gave us a picture of Hunter at a club which met at the British Coffee House: 'Hunter was gay and lively to the last degree, and often came in to us at 9 o'clock fatigued and jaded. He had no dinner, but supped on a couple of eggs and drank his glass of claret; for though we were a punch club, we allowed him a bottle of what he liked best. He repaid us with the brilliancy of his conversation. His toast was "May no English nobleman venture out of the world without a Scottish physician, as I am sure there is none who ventures in!"'.

In his later years all Hunter's spare time was taken up with the formation of his vast collection of books[40], coins, pictures, minerals and objects of natural history.[41] When he died in 1783 he left his museum and £8,000 to Glasgow University with the condition attached that it was to remain in London for the use of his partner Cruikshank and his nephew, Matthew Baillie, for thirty years. Baillie in 1802 intimated to the University of Glasgow that he was now ready to give up the museum whenever Glasgow had a building fit to receive it. An elegant classical building was erected in the gardens of the University and was completed in 1807. In 1870 the contents of the museum were relocated in the new University buildings at Gilmorehill.

Hunter's lasting scientific fame rests on his contributions to reproductive anatomy and physiology, but he also had an immense influence as a teacher of clinical obstetrics. In clear, pungent phrases he stressed again and again the dangers of unnecessary intervention and the advantages of leaving normal labour to nature. 'If I were allowed to give an account of myself I may say that I had never been of more service to mankind than in making this my practice and advice' he pronounced, adding that 'the great art in conducting a natural labour is to do little, and wait patiently'.[42]

This conservative teaching was followed in the great obstetric textbooks of subsequent generations such as those of Denman[43] and Ramsbotham[44]. But Newton's first law applies to medicine as well as to physics. To every action there is a reaction, and the late 19th century saw a revival of interventionist obstetrics, culminating in the development of Caesarean section. Nonetheless, modern obstetrics rests firmly on the rational foundation laid in the 18th century by the three London Scots, practising 'furth of Scotland', with whom this essay deals. These man-midwives were not mere technical experts; they were men of science and men of letters, true sons of the Enlightenment, in whom the faculties of wonder and of reason were both highly developed.

Acknowledgements

I am grateful to Mr Phillip Escreet and Dr Nigel Thorp of the Special Collections Department, Glasgow University Library, and to Mr Martin Hopkinson of the Hunterian Art Gallery for help in my study of original material relating to Hunter and Douglas. Mr Ralph Winterton gave me access to the early records of the Middlesex Hospital. Mr Alex Rodger, Librarian, Royal College of Physicians and Surgeons of Glasgow and Dr Derek Dow, Archivist, Greater Glasgow Health Board, also gave me helpful advice.

The Irish Connection

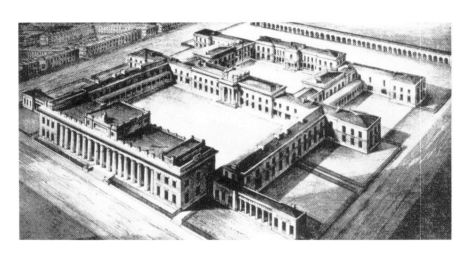

Sir John Soane's ambitious plans for The Royal Belfast Academical Institution, 1809. In the event only one of the three proposed blocks could be funded at this time.

Chapter 5

The Irish Connection

P Froggatt

Prologue

Nowhere has Scottish medicine in its ideas, practices, and the influence of its graduates, been more seminal and ubiquitous than in the northern half of Ireland. In this paper I explain why this should be, describe the foundation (in 1835) of the 'Belfast medical school' which avidly embraced Scottish educational and medical practices, and note that this direct Scottish influence waned after about 1850 though even today it remains a most respected and influential exotic professional and academic force. I will finish with the eclipse in 1849 of this early school by The Queen's University in Ireland – a new creation conceived in London and Dublin Castle and forged at Westminster in an effort to meet demand for university education for all Irishmen irrespective of creed who could avail themselves of it, or (to the cynic) to woo the now enfranchised Irish Catholic middle classes away from opposing the Union! I will assume that the commonality of culture between Ulster and Scotland, which had ancient origins, enjoyed periodic re-enrichments and provided a ready-made seeding-bed for the medical practices which Ulstermen imported from Scotland, is well-known and needs neither emphasis nor explanation.

Background

The medical school of Trinity College Dublin (hereinafter Trinity) was the first in Ireland: though founded in 1711 it only offered a coherent system of instruction, and that haphazard, after 1786 (and in practice a generation later) when it was united by Act of Parliament with the Royal College of Physicians of Ireland. The latter drew much vigour, inspiration and (more surprisingly perhaps) actual specie from an expatriot Aberdonian, Sir Patrick Dun, thus ensuring an early Scottish influence on the Irish medical stage.[1] Trinity and the Guild of Barber-Surgeons followed contemporary penal practices against Catholics and they were forced to study abroad — mainly in France and Italy where cultural and religious empathy and often political affinities were conducive.[2] Some Protestants did likewise: Hans Sloane, of Chelsea Gardens fame, took his degree at the University in Orange (a town near Avignon in the department of Vaucluse), a long way from his humble childhood in Killyleagh, Co. Down, a village which shares with Inverness the favour of a subsidiary title for the Duke of York![3] But things in Ireland are not always what they seem: some Catholics became prudential converts to Anglicanism and benefited materially (including facility of educational opportunity) as a recompense for any spiritual debasement with the convenient option of becoming reconciled to the Old Religion as judgement day approached.[4]

Despite penal rigours it was not among the predominantly Catholic population that the iniquities of educational disabilities first became an issue but among another more localised majority — Dissenters, mainly Presbyterians of Scottish extraction in Belfast, Down and Antrim. They also suffered penalties, though less harsh than those of Catholics, but unlike Catholics they were becoming an increasingly prosperous and upwardly mobile group — intellectually restless, politically questioning and much influenced by the Scottish Enlightenment and events in America and France. All but four of the sixty-five or so founder members of the Belfast Chamber of Commerce in 1784 were Presbyterians,[5] while throughout eastern Ulster and in parts of western Ulster also, they constituted an extensive reticulum of rural tenants, agrarian merchants, general tradesmen, farmers, and a literate coterie of doctors, notaries, and clergy. They wished their sons to improve themselves beyond harvest-field, counting-house and high stool, and would brook no bar to these ambitions, but they were denied the traditional patronage of local grandee still more of a deeply mistrusting government. Necessity as well as inclination turned many towards medicine and the church, and turned some also to armed rebellion. But the ground was stony. Oxford and Cambridge were closed to them: only Anglicans could matriculate at the former prior to 1854 or graduate at the latter before 1856. Trinity disadvantaged them, no great hindrance perhaps since it existed as a medical school only in name with an average of less than five students per year until the turn of the century.[6] The newly opened (in 1784) school of the

Royal College of Surgeons in Ireland, and the private schools of anatomy and medicine in Dublin, welcomed them, but these would not enjoy their hey-day for a generation or more. In any event the northern Presbyterian viewed Dublin as culturally remote and, worse, expensive and morally dangerous, and London more so. He therefore chose Scotland (predominantly Edinburgh for medicine and Glasgow for arts and divinity) because of its famous and growing schools free of religious test, where his sons could at least sin with co-religionists which presumably made it more acceptable! The thin trickle of Irishmen to Scotland now became something of a flood, and the sons of Ulster merchants, farmers and the manse were familiar passengers on the packet from Donaghadee to Portpatrick en route to study medicine, humanities and divinity. Only detailed research could quantify this exodus; only a Namier-type study could put flesh on the statistical bones. I have so far done neither but thanks to help from Dr Derek Dow, Miss Lesley De Jean and Dr Christine Johnson, I can paint some form of representational rather than impressionistic picture, though it lacks pre-Raphaelite detail. The figures given below are necessarily only a proxy of the actual number of Irish students studying any branch of 'medicine' in Scotland at the time.

The Ulster exodus to Scotland

There were 800 Edinburgh and 170 Glasgow MDs awarded in the last quarter of the 18th century.[7] Of these, 311 (32%) were to Irishmen, which far outstripped the 246 (25%) to English and 218 (22%) to Scottish recipients. This averaged admittedly only some 12 Irish graduates a year but was substantial at a time when Trinity was producing only two or three and Continental school recruitment of Irishmen was affected by the European and revolutionary wars. Even before 1775 Irish students were graduating in Edinburgh though in modest numbers — 56 took the MD in the twenty-seven years from 1748, an average of two a year.[8] Most returned home, some after further study at other centres, and this brought the Scottish and particularly the Edinburgh influence early into Irish practice. The pace quickened at the turn of the century: the population of Ireland was increasing rapidly and nowhere quicker than in largely Presbyterian Belfast;[9] the country was prosperous; and the Napoleanoic War put high demands for medical manpower on all the Kingdom. From 1800 to 1825 there were 1,938 Edinburgh and 256 Glasgow MDs.[10] Again the Irish predominated — 647 (33%) or some 25 per year including such household names as Abraham Colles, William Stokes and Dominic Corrigan, and many others of local eminence or whose fame time has eclipsed. Concomitantly Irish enrolments in Professor James Jeffray's anatomy class in Glasgow rose even more dramatically from about 16 to over 40 per year (24%). In 1813 the total reached 97 and was often over 70.[11] The Edinburgh University anatomy lists, less complete, show an average of some 44 Irish per year (15%) in the decade 1790-1800, falling to 30 per year in 1800-20 in line with the fall in total enrolments: the percentage of 15% remained the same.[12] I leave it to Edinburgh medical historians to explain the overall decline which may have resulted from the deadening effect of the teaching of Alexander Monro (tertius) which is abundantly documented ('Dr. [Monro] made his lectures on human anatomy as dull as he was himself, and the subject disgusted me'[13]) and growing competition from private schools, especially those of John Barclay and, later, Robert Knox; possibly it was other factors. But what happened after about 1815-20 in both Edinburgh and Glasgow is certainly not ambiguous: both the proportion and absolute number of Irish *anatomy* students, though not necessarily *medical* students, fell markedly. 'I should think,' Jeffray told the Scottish University Commissioners in 1827, 'that the [Irish] medical students have diminished in some respect because more go now to Dublin and Paris etc. where they get the [anatomical] subjects much easier than we are able to procure them here'.[14] This refers to the burgeoning schools in Dublin after about 1810 (which I have mentioned) and to the difficulties encountered by Scottish resurrection-ists despite the importing of their wares from Ireland and the activities of my two compatriots, James Burke and William Hare, who tried in a rather personal way to reciprocate to Scottish medical education for what Scottish medical education undoubtedly contributed to Ireland! Jeffray went on to claim that: 'The academy at Belfast has also lessened our numbers'. It is to this so-called 'academy at Belfast' that I now turn.

The Ulster answer: an independent medical school in Belfast

Irish students in Scotland were predominantly Presbyterians from Ulster. As a sample, Jeffray's class list for 1820-1 shows 27 Irish students. The provenance of 22 is recorded: all but one were from Ulster. Most of the names recorded were almost certainly Presbyterian though some possibly belonged to other dissenting sects or were Anglicans. None had a characteristic aboriginal or Catholic name.

Over half were from Antrim or Down, counties with large Presbyterian majorities. The class list of five years later confirms these biases.
The Irish on the Edinburgh University anatomy rolls were of wider
provenance with sprinklings from southern counties, but there is still
a clear northern preponderance.

This substantial and growing exodus of Ulster's sons did not go
unnoticed. A local university without religious test was needed; Ireland
after all had twice the population of Scotland, though was something
of a witches' brew of religious affiliations correlated with political
advantages. One was planned for Armagh, the Primatial capital, and
Primate Robinson willed some handsome buildings and £5,000 in 1796
to endow it. His dead hand was to hold the purse since the offer was
to lapse after five years.[15] His hopes were blown away with the
gunsmoke of the 1798 rebellion. Presbyterians now took up the running
and conceived a composite 'Academical Institution'[16] to provide
schooling for their younger sons, collegiate instruction in arts and
medicine for their older ones, and continuing education — described in
the 1808 Prospectus as 'popular lectures upon those subjects which are
most conducive to the improvement of the Agriculture, Arts and
Manufacture of the country . . . [with] a Library and Museum for
fossils, models of useful instruments and machines and engines . . . and
natural curiosities'.[17] In short, a Scottish university in embryo with a
school and extramural department tacked on. Dr William Drennan, a
founder of the Society of United Irishmen and author of their
constitution, and an Edinburgh MD of 1778, in his opening address on
1 February 1814 underscored the exodus of young talent:

> '[The Institution's objects are] . . . to diffuse as widely as possible through the
> province and population of Ulster, the benefits of Education both useful and
> liberal; and by that means to prevent the hard and disgraceful necessity, in such
> a great and prosperous community, of sending their children to seek in other
> countries, with much risk to their health and morals, for that instruction . . .
> which might be equally attained at home . . . with evident advantage to the
> public interest as well as to that of individuals'.[18]

This Institution was incorporated by Act of Parliament in 1810 as
a non-denominational foundation though with a strong Presbyterian
ethos — secular education taken in common; religious education
separately; self-improvement, diligence, providence, and self-control
the cardinal virtues; and an evangelical commitment which assumed
that attaining goods in this world and salvation in the next would be
the joint rewards of virtue! The uncompromising slogan on prize
medals was 'work is everything', the school motto was, and is, 'seek

the truth'. On 1 November 1815 'Inst' — as it is still called — opened its collegiate doors to a few dozen students who would otherwise have boarded the packet to Scotland. The general certificate course was recognised by the General (Presbyterian) Synod of Ulster as equivalent to a Scottish MA, and even supported by the unrelenting 'subscription-ist' Presbyterian Synod of Ireland — usually called Seceders — giving a grand total of over 300 Presbyterian congregations.

The founders also planned a medical school.[19] There was already a Professor of Natural Philosophy — Andrew Ure of Glasgow, a Glasgow MD of 1801 and lecturer in chemistry at Glasgow's Andersonian University. Additional chairs of chemistry, botany, and anatomy and human physiology were high on the priority list as were plans for a four-room anatomy suite and an adjoining botanical garden, while several clinical chairs were to be created after discussions with the Fever Hospital (later the General Hospital and now The Royal Victoria Hospital, Belfast). But their hopes were dashed. Three staff and five members of the joint board of managers and visitors were reported drinking seditious toasts at a St Patrick's Day banquet in 1816 ('to Marshal Ney', '14th July' and 'reform of the franchise' are examples). Despite disciplinary action and avowals of loyalty by Inst, government withdrew its grant of £1,500 p.a. in the event for thirteen long years. Plans for the medical school were reluctantly shelved but three years later Dr James Lawson Drummond, a native of Ballyclare, Co. Antrim, and an Edinburgh MD of 1814, started lectures in anatomy and physiology at £50 salary. His class consisted largely of theology students but also included some students of medicine: 'I teach a very wide field of natural history and a good deal of natural theology: there is scarcely a fact in Paley's *Natural Theology* that is not explained and illustrated . . . [also] a little human dissection'.[20] He added a course in botany in 1822 and was enrolling in his classes as many as 26 students by the time Jeffray was rather exaggeratedly if accurately bewailing to the Scottish Universities Commissioners that 'The Academy at Belfast has also lessened our numbers'.

The next dozen years were ones of frustration and only piece-meal progress, Without its grant Inst teetered perenially on the brink of bankruptcy. Wages were slashed and salaries halved, including that of the stipendiary secretary — Robert Simms, a republican United Irishman hero of 1798 who for the cause had sampled the Scottish breezes of Fort George during His Majesty's pleasure. Maintenance was deferred, purchases cancelled or postponed and expansion aborted, including the plans for a department of medicine. In contrast, Inst's prospective partner — the General Hospital — enjoyed comparatively halcyon days. Its new 110-bed hospital opened in 1817, students walked the wards from 1820, and from 1827 an identifiable if somewhat uncertain series of clinical lectures was inaugurated by the doyen of Ulster medicine, Dr James McDonnell, erstwhile friend and host of the arch-republication Wolfe Tone, and an Edinburgh MD of 1784. In 1827 the horizon lightened — the Irish Education Commissioners recommended that Inst's grant be restored and it was now only a matter of time until a joint Inst/General Hospital school could be created under Inst's control. Common purpose, regional need, local pride, provincial cohesion, and overlapping membership of the committee and staff of the General Hospital and the joint board of managers and visitors of Inst, inevitable in such a tight-knit community (Drummond was formerly consultant physician to the Hospital as well as the incumbent of two chairs at Inst, and there were other examples) ensured the ends. The means, however, were to present many problems as the profession fought for overall control, as professions will, but in the end the Inst proprietors proved immovable on fundamentals while comprising on detail. The medical fraternity were at last wooed from their pursuit of the Harlot's Prerogative, and finally, on 8 October 1835, the 'Board of Faculty of the Medical Department of the Royal Belfast Academical Institution' held its first meeting with five of its planned twelve professors in post, James Lawson Drummond as Dean, an enlightened curriculum accepted of a four year joint pre-clinical and clinical course, a complete system of study, examination, discipline and procedure published, and students shortly to be enrolled. The school was firmly governed by Inst and free from hospital staff control — unlike provincial schools in England and Dublin; free from town council control — unlike Edinburgh; and free from undue influence of professional bodies — unlike Glasgow and Trinity. It was in essence a partnership between an incorporated autonomous multitechnic college and a voluntary hospital though firmly subordinate to the college statutes — a structural prototype (barring some niceties) of the modern medical school. It was arguably the most perfectly structured of any school outside the national capitals of the Kingdom, and perhaps inside them also!

Progress of the school

Each of the five foundation medical professors held a Scottish MD:

James Drummond (anatomy and physiology, and botany) of Edinburgh 1814; John McDonnell (surgery), James's son, of Edinburgh 1825 in a class which included William Stokes and Dominic Corrigan; Thomas Andrews (chemistry) of Edinburgh 1835; James Drummond Marshall (materia medica and pharmacy) of Edinburgh 1831; the fifth, Robert Little (midwifery and diseases of women and children), ventured closer to the Ailsa Craig which he could see from his attic bedroom near Ballywalter on the Ards coast and took the Glasgow MD in 1826.[21] Henry MacCormac was appointed to the combined chair of the theory and practice of physic in 1837: he was an Edinburgh MD of 1824 and father of Sir William MacCormac, Bt., first Irishman to be President of the Royal College of Surgeons of England (1896-1901).[22] Robert Coffey who succeeded to the chair of surgery in 1837 was MD Glasgow of 1833, and with even the demonstrator in anatomy a Scottish graduate — James Sanders, MD Edinburgh of 1835 — the entire faculty and its single medical surrogate were a solid clique of Scottish graduates. So were most of the physicians to the hospital and many of the surgeons, including those who gave the clinical lectures. The parchments of, as distinct from study at, Dublin or London or Continental Europe were unfamiliar commodities among the Ulster medical fraternity of the time.

The curriculum not surprisingly was based on Scottish practice, not in its pristine form but blended with that distillation of Scottish and best Continental methods introduced to the Meath Hospital by Robert Graves in 1821,[23] and disseminated among a wide and growing studentship by the glittering coterie of eminent physicians which characterised the high noon of Dublin medicine. Many of the Belfast leaders studied in Dublin before completing in Scotland — Andrews, McDonnell, MacCormac, Little, and Sanders are cases in point — and so drank not just deeply but twice over at the Pierian spring of Scottish/Dublin medical practice. This is not the place to describe the principles of the Edinburgh and Dublin methods which by the early 19th century had crucial dissimilarities[24], but teaching in Belfast was characterised by meticulous case-notes, emphasis on clinical signs and clinical diagnosis, the relating of autopsy findings to clinical disease, emphasis on the physical over the symptomatic, operative surgical instruction, and close involvement of students in bedside diagnosis and care. Small wonder that with all this on the doorstep and Belfast burgeoning in size and wealth, the school thrived and in its fourteen years averaged 50 students per year with over 100 subject enrolments and nearly twice that in the peak years of the early 1840s. This placed it among the larger provincial schools — equal to Bristol and Jordan's school in Manchester, smaller than Birmingham and the Royal school, Manchester, but larger than Liverpool, York, Newcastle and possibly Leeds.[25] When to this is added the fame and facilities of contemporary Dublin medicine, a greater tolerance of the capital's supposedly wicked ways by a more cosmopolitan and certainly more affluent Ulster population, and the end of the grossest anti-papist discriminations, then the decline of Irish students and graduands in Scotland by the 1830s, so lamented by Jeffray, is entirely explicable in domestic Irish terms without appeal to coeval events in Scotland which militated against the popularity of the Scottish schools.

The new Belfast school at once sought recognition for its courses. The Faculty of Physicians and Surgeons of Glasgow and the Royal College of Surgeons of Edinburgh quickly complied, as did the University of St Andrews. The Universities of Edinburgh and Aberdeen were not approached. Glasgow University was, but had clearly a longer memory as well as a greater vested interest. Inst vigorously pursued the matter but without success. The first approach in August 1836 drew the reply that 'the University was quite opposed to the recognition of any new medical schools' and would not accept the Inst certificate 'as part of the qualification of candidates for medicine and surgery honours at Glasgow University'. Inst now tried reassurance, and offered to confirm to the University 'that students in Belfast would only be induced to attend our lectures for a season or two preparatory to studying in Glasgow, instead of going, as they now usually do, to the South of Ireland' — a reference to Inst's *raison dêtre* and to the recent but now waning popularity of the classes in anatomy and surgery in Trinity under the legendary James Macartney who at his peak had regularly enrolled up to 90 students annually.[26] Glasgow University, however, were not only opposed to recognising Inst, they seemed also opposed to answering Inst's letters and subsequent approaches lay ignored, the last one being as late as 14 April 1843. Glasgow had benefited most from the Ulster exodus and stood to lose most when it waned. The University had tried hard to preserve it and even introduced a two-level degree in surgery in 1819 to remain competitive: indeed, all seven students who took the new Bachelor's as distinct from Master's degree were Irish. The ChB was discontinued in 1822, but undoubtedly Glasgow felt the loss of its Irish student regiments.[27]

The early 1840s marked Inst's zenith. The cause of its decline ironically lay not with medicine but elsewhere. The schism in the Ulster Presbyterian Church over the Arian heterodoxies encouraged the General Synod (and *a fortiori* the Seceders) to withdraw their recognition of licentiates from the Inst faculty of arts as being allegedly tainted with 'new light' propaganda, and this rubbed off on the sister faculty of medicine. Secondly, in 1845 government decreed that a new non-denominational university — The Queen's University in Ireland — with colleges in Belfast, Cork, and Galway should be formed to encourage non-denominational tertiary education. This was intended to dissuade the sons of the now emancipated and burgeoning Catholic majority from studying in Catholic (i.e. nationalist) establishments in Ireland, or, worse, so-called 'democratic' institutions in Europe and America which would instill seditious (i.e. anti-Union) ideas. This double blow floored Inst as a college and in 1849 the Inst medical school closed and the students transferred to the new Queen's College Belfast, and from that day most Ulster students sought the degrees of the new Queen's University in Ireland rather than those of Edinburgh or Glasgow. The decline of Irish emigrants for Scottish degrees accelerated: the historic 30% of Irish in each Edinburgh MD class had dropped to 14% in the 1840s. By 1855 it had halved again, and by 1860 numbered only three individuals.[28] The classes themselves had greatly reduced in number for reasons which students of Edinburgh medicine will know well.[29]

Ironically Inst lost its school as events were moving in its favour: the new 600-bed Union Fever Hospital opened in 1849 — this meant better clinical material in the General Hospital; the Belfast Dispensary was reorganised; and Andrew Malcolm, the unsung genius of Belfast medicine, hardly known because of his early death at 38, returned to Belfast in 1842 with his Edinburgh MD in his pocket and in his head and heart a resolve to reaffirm Belfast's commitment to its Scottish mentors and to its charitable traditions so sorely distorted by the new industrial wealth.[30] However, it was all too late for Inst. Queen's reaped the benefits, but as the Ulster medical fraternity now started to change from one of Scottish graduates to one mainly of Irish ones they remained the heirs to an 18th century Scottish medical and educational tradition which itself reached back to Leyden and Boerhaave. Just as all the early professors in 19th century Belfast were Edinburgh graduates (save only Robert Little and Robert Coffey — and they were Glasgow men) so the first five professors in the new

Edinburgh faculty after 1726 had studied at Leyden between 1718 and
1722 when Boerhaave was at his peak.[31] The enrichments, dilutions and
perhaps vulgarisation of the Scottish medical experience in Ulster as
it has passed through two centuries of Irish practice, even though
seeded on a Scots-Irish Ulster substrate and influenced by not a little
English and American input this century, is a fertile field for further
study which has been no more than cursorily examined.[32]

Epilogue

Ulster medicine has distinctive characteristics which can be identified
largely unchanged over nearly two centuries. In its *practice*, it is the
heir to a pragmatic and clinically orientated tradition whose genesis
lies in the sense of values of the Ulster society which spawned it and
which produced the bulk of Ulster's doctors. This society required
practical abilities and provided the robust, puritan, and unsophisticated
milieu of a rural, even frontier people. It had little time for
philosophising, still less for acquiring metropolitan graces. Clinical,
ethical and educative commitment have been high; research achievements less notable, due more to a certain rugged individualism which
has not been conducive to development of that large-scale team work
which now dictates success than to any lack of interest in intellectual
inquiry. In its adherence to the *tradition* of the profession it has
emphasised teaching, an enthusiasm based on high rectitude and the
tenets of Presbyterianism which until recently have been powerful
determinants of the Ulster profession's attitudes, and teaching a
method grounded in Graves's procedures of observation at the bedside.
In its *compassion* and *commitment* it draws not just on ethical but on the
common cultural and historical identity between doctor and patient —
Ulster's doctors were never Pall Mall gentlemen owing their
physician's rank to high birth or their surgical advancement to crude
patronage or nepotism, and they identified fully with their patients.
Above all, the Ulster profession is both *coherent* and *cohesive*, an
inescapable consequence of the fact that in our whole history the great
majority of students, general practitioners and their professional
forebears, and, until the last thirty years or so, hospital clinical staff
also have been Ulstermen and women. In-breeding can be vitiating and
has certainly helped to shape the profession's characteristics in a fairly
inflexible mould, but the mould has been a good one and in fact there
has always been enough importation to ensure hybrid vigour.

Many of these characteristics are shared with Scottish medicine; it has been a purpose of this paper to bring some of the basic facts of the 'Irish connection' to the readers of the symposium.

Scottish Doctors and the English Public Health

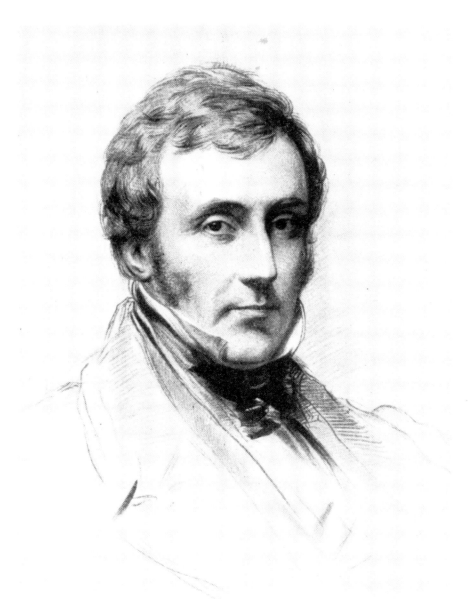

William Pulteney Alison (1790-1859), a dominant figure in the emergent public health debate both north and south of the border.

Chapter 6
Scottish Doctors and the English Public Health
B White

To remove doubt as to what constitutes a SCOTTISH DOCTOR, for the purposes of this paper it pertains to those doctors whose medical degrees and diplomas were gained from Scottish medical institutions: though, to paraphrase a well known saying, this may well involve some doctors having Scottishness thrust upon them.

Some of the leading figures in English public health history were products of a Scottish medical education. The link between the men and the discipline is neither tenuous nor fleeting. It is substantial and lasted, for the purposes of this paper, throughout the 19th century.

The strong presence of Scottish doctors surrounding Chadwick's sanitary endeavours in the 1830s and 1840s cannot have escaped the notice of those interested in the history of social medicine. The three medical reporters for the Poor Law Commissioners in the 1839 enquiry into sanitary measures to check the course of fever in London were all Scottish graduates: Southwood Smith and James Phillips Kay were Edinburgh MDs; Neil Arnott was an Aberdeen MD. Their reports led to Chadwick's comprehensive investigation into the Sanitary Condition of the Labouring Population of Great Britain, completed in 1842. This in turn precipitated the statutory enactments of 1847-8, culminating in the 1848 Public Health Act for England and Wales. The Act's main features were the introduction of local authority medical officers of health and the formation of a General Board of Health.

The Metropolitan Health of Towns Association, formed after Chadwick's Report and the vanguard of sanitary improvement agitation, had a fair sprinkling of Scottish graduates including George Milroy, John Sutherland and Hector Gavin, all of whom later joined the General Board of Health — Gavin as a medical inspector, Sutherland as one of the Board's two medical superintending inspectors and Milroy as Superintendent General of medical inspectors. Their appointments at the General Board of Health make an interesting constellation when matched with Southwood Smith as the Board's medical member, for only Sutherland was an Aberdeen MD; the others were all from Edinburgh. Almost like the three musketeers, Gavin, Milroy and Sutherland were also members of the Sanitary Commission sent to the Crimea and headed by Sutherland.[1] Their task was no doubt facilitated by the director of the Army's medical statistics department, Surgeon General TG Balfour, MD Edinburgh, and their findings were perhaps acted upon by the Army Medical Inspector of Hospitals (Sanitary Branch), TG Logan, a licentiate of the Royal College of Surgeons of Edinburgh in 1827 and MD Glasgow 1838. If, on their return from the Crimea the commissioners had anything in their baggage approaching contraband status they might have called upon the help of the Customs Board MOH, James McWilliam Ormiston, MD Edinburgh 1840, FRCS Edinburgh 1857, and author of several government papers on cholera and yellow fever . . .

Of the Metropolitan MOHs appointed in 1855 only three held Scottish degrees. The most outstanding of them was John Burdon Sanderson, MD Edinburgh 1851, lecturer in medical jurisprudence at St Mary's Hospital and medical inspector for the Privy Council's department of health under John Simon. Sanderson later became Waynefleete Professor of Physiology at Oxford.[2]

Between 1848 and 1855 some thirty-nine provincial towns in England and Wales appointed MOHs and of these thirteen held Scottish qualifications.[3] However, the predominance of Edinburgh graduates becomes almost overpowering when transferred to Liverpool's public health history. Liverpool has the distinction of appointing the first-ever MOH in Britain in 1847 under the local Liverpool Improvement Act. Their MOH was Henry Duncan, a native Liverpudlian with an Edinburgh MD. Duncan's successor was William Trench, his contemporary and fellow student. In 1878 Trench was followed by John Stopford Taylor, LRCP Edinburgh and MD Aberdeen. In 1896 Taylor was followed by Edward Hope, MD Edinburgh. This gave Liverpool an unbroken run of almost eighty years of MOHs holding Scottish qualifications. The Edinburgh-Liverpool nexus possibly sprang from Thomas S Traill, MD Edinburgh 1802, a local practitioner and lecturer, who was appointed the fourth Regius Professor of Medical Jurisprudence and Medical Police at Edinburgh in 1833.

Why did graduates of the Scottish universities and medical licensing corporations appear to figure so prominently in the initial period of English public health? There seems to be no major binding link other than their medical education. Not all of them were Scots-born. Not all of them were from the Protestant dissenting community. Few of them had medical backgrounds. For instance Arnott came from Scottish Catholic farming stock, Kay from a Rochdale banking and legal family, Southwood Smith was a Unitarian minister, and Henry Duncan was a Liverpool merchant's son.[4]

Scottish medical education has a long tradition of public health related teaching stretching back to the end of the 18th century under its older title of 'medical police'. It was taught under the general heading of medical jurisprudence. This subject comprehended the components of legal or State medicine, namely forensic medicine and medical police. It was a direct European concept imported into Scotland by Andrew Duncan, Professor of Physiology at Edinburgh University, and it owed much to the questioning of man's relationship to the State contained in European *Enlightenment* thought. Bearing in mind that the main theme of the 1986 Edinburgh Festival is *The Scottish Enlightment* it seems churlish not to mention this point.

In the closing decade of the 18th century Duncan included lectures, firstly on forensic medicine then on medical police, into his physiology course. In 1806 he was instrumental in the foundation at Edinburgh of the first Regius chair of medical jurisprudence and medical police in Britain. His son, Andrew Duncan junior, was the first professor. In both medical and political terms it was a radical chair. Because of its connections with revolutionary France (where such chairs were already founded) and with the Whig political cause, the Edinburgh chair was rejected by the Medical Faculty and spent the first years of its life within the Law Faculty. There it enjoyed the protection of the influential Erskine family and withstood Tory attempts to discontinue it.[5]

Under Andrew Duncan, the teaching of medical police developed a peculiarly *Scottish* identity. It covered a wide spectrum of medical provisions and was never tied solely to environmental sanitary improvements as it proved in England. It eschewed State intervention and advocated philanthropic provision by doctors and laymen alike. Philanthropy was charged with applying hospital and dispensary care for the whole range of human needs from the cradle to the grave. Doctors were instructed in contagious and epidemic disease and the basic elementary principles of hygiene – air, water, food, drink, clothing, occupations and salubrious places for siting towns. It retained this wide-ranging interpretation well into the second half of the 19th century.

Whereas medical police taught on matters affecting the health or comfort of individuals and on sanitary regulations affecting the health of communities, its major partner, forensic medicine, dealt with matters affecting the civil and social rights of individuals. It is important to note that in Scotland the two were taught in tandem throughout the 19th century. Furthermore, as the teaching of forensic medicine and medical police spread to Glagow and Aberdeen, these subjects became mandatory elements for licentiates of the Scottish medical corporations (from 1832) and for Scottish university medical graduates (from 1833). Thus, after 1833, Scottish trained doctors had the distinct advantage of having compulsory academic instruction on those points of medicine where it came in contact with the law.

In England the position was quite different. The coupling of forensic medicine and public health as academic subjects never gained much ground. Although most London and provincial medical schools taught forensic medicine by the mid century, by 1878 there remained difficulties in having it accepted as an examinable subject in its own right.[6] It is interesting to note that although medical police lectures were given in some medical schools, according to John Simon the first *public health* lectures given in England were delivered in London, at St Thomas's in 1856 by Edward Greenhow.[7] Dr Greenhow graduated MD Aberdeen in 1814.

Apart from Andrew Duncan, the major figure associated with the teaching of medical police in Scotland was William Pulteney Alison. Alison was the second Regius Professor of the subjects at Edinburgh for a little over two years from 1819-21, after which he became successively Professor of Physiology then of Medicine. As Professor of Medical Jurisprudence and Medical Police, Alison retained Duncan's philanthropic ethos. He thought there were two ways to promote the public health, either by framing positive laws or by medical men actively persuading people to attend to existing regulations by pointing out the consequences of omission. Alison preferred persuasion. He thought municipal public health enactments infringed the liberty and comforts of the individual and could only be justified when existing enactments proved totally inadequate.[8] Alison never lost interest in medical police and continued to include some part of it in his later teaching. His work at the Edinburgh New Dispensary brought him intimate contact with Edinburgh's poor and the incidence of typhus, typhoid and smallpox, an experience reflected in his teachings.

The majority of doctors named earlier in this paper were Alison's pupils. Kay was chosen by Alison to work in the New Dispensary during a typhus epidemic while he was still a student. When, after 1833, forensic medicine and medical police became compulsory for medical degrees at Edinburgh, those who graduated had necessarily attended Traill's course of lectures on forensic medicine and medical police in addition to Alison's lectures in medicine, or had attended extra-mural lectures. It was a formidable combination for those graduates who either went south to seek their fortunes or returned there after studying for a degree. If there was a seemingly high incidence of Scottish graduates involved in the initial years of English public health, their interest may well have been influenced by such factors. Certainly the Army and Navy Boards recommended medical jurisprudence by the 1830s and in Scotland this included medical police. But it must not be forgotten that in general the early MOHs were often very poorly paid and equally poorly regarded. Struggling young Scottish doctors practising in England had perforce to capitalise on their public health knowledge by taking the opportunities frowned on by more established practitioners.

It must be one of the great ironies of public health history that Alison's pupils figured so prominently during the early period of English public health. Edwin Chadwick and his medical followers disagreed emphatically with Alison on such fundamental issues as the etiology of disease and legal enactments to control public health. Put in simple terms, English public health efforts under Chadwick espoused the miasmatic theory and its relationship of dirt-to-disease-leading-to-destitution. Alison believed implicitly in the contagion theory, quarantine, and the predisposing factor of destitution as a major influence in the spread of fevers. Contemporary public rhetoric in Scotland, led by Alison, centred not on public health reform but on an enhanced Poor Law to alleviate destitution and so reduce the underlying causes of disease. These mid 19th century interpretations of the etiology of disease serve to emphasise that English and Scottish customs differed on such relevant details as housing, Poor Law administration and local government sanitary provision.

The gulf separating the two camps became painfully clear when Chadwick's Report was published in 1842. It included Alison's

Observations on the generation of Fever and Arnott's report *On the Fevers which have prevailed in Edinburgh and Glasgow*, both of which appeared to set Edinburgh and London on a collision course. At Chadwick's General Board of Health the value of quarantine was questioned when cholera threatened in 1848: Milroy had already written the pamphlet *Cholera not be arrested by quarantine*. In Liverpool, Henry Duncan firmly believed, amongst other things, that air contaminated by rotting vegetable matter brought disease.

With these differences, Alison, not surprisingly, organised Scottish medical opposition against Chadwick and successfully thwarted Chadwick's efforts to have similar public health legislation passed to cover Scotland. By adopting this stance Alison rejected the many former students engaged in English public health who had deviated so obviously from his teachings. This painful episode left visible scars. The term 'public health' never received even tentative approval in Edinburgh medical circles until after Alison's death in 1855. The first medical officers of health were not appointed in Scotland until 1862, and even then they were not the result of a Public Health Act, but came under local and general Police Acts.

But Scottish medical degrees and English public health continued to exercise their mutual attraction well into the last quarter of the 19th century. A quick check on MOHs listed in the *Medical Directory* for 1871, just prior to the 1872 Public Health Act which made the appointment of MOHs nominally compulsory in England and Wales, revealed that out of 113 local authority MOHs, 42 of them, or just over 37%, held Scottish medical qualifications.

The public health related legislation passed in the 1870s to cover England and Wales promoted the employment of MOHs and had a noticeable effect on the Scottish medical curriculum. Again Edinburgh dominated the scene. In 1875 the university instituted the science-based degrees of BSc and DSc in public health, open only to medical graduates of recognised universities. Douglas Maclagan, Professor of Forensic Medicine and Public Health, taught the public health courses at undergraduate and postgraduate level and did so with an undeniably English emphasis. Lectures were built around a framework of public health related legislation applicable to England which had no parallel in Scotland. It must be stated that Scottish legal enactments offered little scope for the enhancement of MOHs working in Scotland until the Scottish Local Government Act of 1889.

Edinburgh postgraduate degrees were rigorous, prestigious, and popular with local and central government medical officials alike. This tendency was enhanced when the 1888 and 1889 Local Government Acts relating to England and Scotland demanded that MOHs of large counties must hold one of the public health postgraduate qualifications listed under section 21 of the 1886 Medical Act. Amongst a group of eminent doctors holding the Edinburgh postgraduate BSc and DSc degrees were Frederick Barry of the Local Government Board, John Frederick Sykes, President of the Incorporated Society of Medical Officers of Health and lecturer at Guy's, and Edward Hope of Liverpool.

Quite apart from the university provision, Henry Duncan Littlejohn taught forensic medicine and public health at the Edinburgh extra-mural school within Surgeon's Hall before succeeding Maclagan as Professor of Forensic Medicine. At the Glasgow Royal Infirmary medical school John Glaister, more renowned in later years for his forensic expertise in the course of law, built up a public health laboratory of sufficient standard to be recognised as giving tuition suitable for candidates for the Cambridge Diploma of Public Health.[9] Scottish DPHs given by the Edinburgh and Glasgow Colleges proved popular qualifications for many English medical officers of health.

Summing up the role of Scottish doctors and the English public health one sees that the major influences lay with Edinburgh and its formal introduction in 1806 of medical police teaching in tandem with forensic medicine under the general title of medical jurisprudence. This set the pattern for Scottish medical degrees and diplomas from 1832 onwards. Not all the doctors who held Scottish qualifications and were involved with the English public health movement were Scottish, which suggests that choice took them north of the Border. Once there, especially at Edinburgh, the combined compulsory teaching of medical police with forensic medicine and the concern shown for the subject by the influential figure of William Pulteney Alison tended to encourage student interest. This interest found expression in the English public health movement's emphasis on sanitary control of the environment rather than the Scottish interpretation of disease causation linked to the amelioration of the destitute classes. By the last quarter of the 19th century Scottish medical teaching of public health changed direction and became responsive to the needs of English public health legislation and the growing professionalisation of medical officers of health. In doing so it indirectly fostered the interests of Scottish MOHs. But that is entirely the subject of another paper.

The Scottish Missionary Doctor

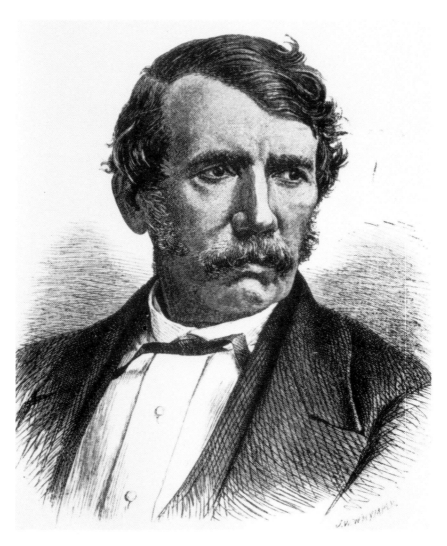

Dr David Livingstone (1813-73).

Chapter 7
The Scottish Missionary Doctor
A C Ross

The Christian religion has, from its beginning, been a missionary faith which seeks to cross cultural as well as geographical frontiers. The 'Letters of Paul' and 'The Acts of the Apostles', which make up a large part of the New Testament, are the story and in some measure the means by which a semitic faith about Jesus of Nazareth being the Messiah was interpreted to the Graeco-Roman world and translated into concepts intelligible within that new cultural framework. Successive waves of missionary effort took this faith to the German and Gaelic tribes beyond the Roman frontiers. Here in Scotland we remember particularly Columba of Derry and Iona, who brought the Christian faith to his fellow Gaels in Scotland; from their new base in Lindisfarne his successors took it to the Germanic tribes who had come to occupy what is now England. The medieval church was a missionary church and in the period of the Reformation the old Church, now designated the Roman Catholic Church, sent forth a new wave of missions spearheaded by a new religious order, the Jesuits, but well supported also by the existing orders, especially the Franciscans and Dominicans. These carried their message into Latin America, India, Indonesia, the Phillipines, Japan and China. On the other side, Protestantism was very unmissionary until what is called in Britain 'The Evangelical Revival', and in America 'The Great Awakening', took place in the middle decades of the 18th century. This transformed the situation of Protestant Christianity in the Netherlands, North America and the United Kingdom particularly. One of the products of the movement was the initiation of a massive missionary effort by Protestants to spread the faith throughout the world. This effort coincided with astonishing developments in western medicine and both those movements came together to produce the missionary doctor.

The alliance was not immediate however. Although the missionary effort got into its stride by the 1790s there was no attempt to send out missionary doctors for some time. This was for two main reasons. In the first place medicine was not so impressively effective in the first two decades of the 19th century as it was later to become, despite the advances made in the late 18th century, particularly in the Scottish universities. Perhaps more important was the fact that within Protestant evangelicalism there was a strain of thought that cared little for material things which were held to be clearly distinct from the things of the spirit. Health and welfare in general were not of the spirit in this view. The missionaries' task was to save souls which otherwise would perish or end in the place of damnation; anything which diverted time and energy from this task was not a concern of the missionary though appropriate for the general charitable action of others. As we shall see, this was not the only strain in Protestant evangelicalism, but it was an important one.

In the hundred years between 1860 and 1960 Scottish missionary doctors served in Africa, the Middle East, the Indian sub-continent, the Far East, the Pacific Islands and the countries of the Caribbean and Latin America; for a period they also served in the Canadian frontier areas. It would be quite impossible in a conference paper to present a survey of this multitude of men and women, of their variety of motivation, their particular attitudes to indigenous traditional religion and medicine, how these changed over the years, and so on. This is a major study which has still to be done. What can be done in the compass of this essay is to examine the Scottish missionary doctor in a general way and then look specifically at what are, perhaps, the two most outstanding Scottish missionary doctors in Africa, David Livingstone and Neil MacVicar.

Before doing so, however, it is worth stressing that, in Africa at least, it was the missions that created a prototype modern health service for the African people and kept it going until well into the 20th century, before the colonial governments did anything at all. In South Africa, the richest country on the continent, whose various component provinces had each some form of autonomy from the 1870s onwards, no government health service had any impact on the African population until the provision of substantial grants from the Union government to mission hospitals in the 1930s, but that was only support for what the churches could do and only went as far as their work had reached. There was no other provision. A health service that was government organised and aimed at being nationwide was a slowly developed structure only created in the period after the Second World War.[1]

The American Board of Commissioners for Foreign Missions commissioned the first missionary doctor, Dr Peter Parker, for service in China in 1834. One or two other men, notably Dr Johannes van der Kemp, the pioneer missionary of the London Missionary Society in South Africa, were medically qualified but when they went to their posts they did so as ministers and evangelists and not as medical missionaries. In China, Parker met an East India Company surgeon, a very devout man who, over and above his official duties, had begun a clinic for Chinese people. The two of them in 1838 founded The Medical Missionary Society in China. The constitution of the Society set the standards which were later adopted by the Scottish missionary doctors. The relevant passages in this constitution are:

> 'Heal the sick is our motto, constituting alike the injunction under which we act and the object at which we aim, and which with the blessing of God, we hope to accomplish by means of scientific practice, in the exercise of an unbought and untiring kindness . . .
>
> . . . In our hospitals we require for the patients the same uniform and well-considered attention which are enjoyed in institutions of a similar kind at home.'

In order to persuade the Christian public in Europe and America that this aim was a vital and essential part of the Christian missionary task, Parker, in 1841, set out on an extensive and exhausting tour of Europe and America. It was certainly needed. In 1826 the Scottish missionaries in the Tyumie Valley in the Cape Colony asked the committee in Scotland to send out a minister who was also a fully qualified physician. They insisted that Africans had bodies to be cured as well as souls to be saved. In addition they pointed out that they and their families were also in need of medical care. Their request was refused.[2] Again, even more striking was the fact that Parker's own Society, the American Board, when it appointed two medically qualified ministers to begin their new mission among the Zulu in 1835, insisted that they must see their task as essentially evangelistic and that their medical work must always be subservient to that end.

In Edinburgh Parker's appeal had a profound effect on a number of leading evangelicals, including several professors in the faculty of medicine. They decided to form what was called a Committee of Co-operation, intended to begin training doctors to serve as medical missionaries and to persuade the churches and societies of the need for them. Two years later the Committee changed its name to The Edinburgh Medical Missionary Society.

At first progress was slow along both prongs of the Society's attack. One thing which it did decide was of fundamental importance; those who were to be trained should be of the very highest quality academically and while doing the course in the medical faculty they should also begin, in Scotland, the kind of work they would be called on to do abroad. In order to achieve this end the Committee in 1858 created the Medical Mission Dispensary and Training Institute in the Cowgate, then an appalling and overcrowded slum area. In this Institute the students were to live and work. They were to aid the resident doctors and so gain experience medically but also to help with what we would now call social work and with prayer meetings and Bible study groups. The Society also felt that those sent out after training should be committed to teaching medical skills to indigenous people, at an appropriate level and as soon as possible.

The Society lived up to this ideal itself. The first two men to complete their medical training at Edinburgh under its auspices graduated in 1857, just as the Cowgate project was being planned. They were Dr Daniel H Paterson, who went to India, and Dr Wong Fun who returned to his own land under the auspices of the London Missionary Society. The latter would appear to have been the first Chinese graduate of Edinburgh University. In 1866 a young Armenian from Lebanon went out to Palestine to found the Christian Hospital in Nazareth. PK Vartan was trained in medicine at Edinburgh University and the Cowgate, another Edinburgh University first.

The Edinburgh Medical Missionary Society set a pattern for the understanding of the nature of the role of the missionary doctor which was of profound importance for Scottish missionary doctors. In the Cowgate the candidates were introduced to an understanding of mission which saw the spreading of the Gospel as a matter of preaching, Bible study, healing the sick and injured, and helping the oppressed and downtrodden to achieve a better standard of living and a greater sense of self-worth. Salvation was for the whole person. This was the other strain in the evangelical tradition that came into being with the Great Awakening, the tradition that produced the anti-slavery campaigns in Britain and America. In a little book produced in 1899 to propagate the cause of medical missions, J Rutter

Williamson, a brilliant American missionary doctor trained by Edinburgh University and the EMMS, chose this quotation from William Lloyd Garrison with which to preface a key chapter:

'In the name of God, Who has made us of one blood and in Whose image we are created; in the name of the Messiah, Who came to bind up the broken hearted, to proclaim liberty to the captives and the opening of the prison to them that are bound, I demand the immediate emancipation of those who are pining.'[4]

In the previous decade John Lowe, who headed the EMMS for over thirty years from 1861, wrote in a pious and pompous style but with the same meaning:

'A minister, while visiting in his parish in one of the most destitute and degraded districts of a great city, after ascending a long, dark, winding stair, opened a door leading into a cheerless garret room. There on a pallet of straw, with no covering, save her dirty, tattered garments, lay an aged woman, to all appearances dying. Forgetting, for the moment, her outward circumstances, in his anxiety for the welfare of her soul, he enquired with all earnestness whether she had any hope for the world to come. "Oh, Sir," she said, as she stretched out her naked, withered arm, "if you were as cold and hungry as I am, you could think of nothing else." That servant of God was taught the lesson that, to succeed in the highest aim of christian love, our ministry must contemplate man in the whole extent of his being; that the disciple of Christ, in so far as he imbibes the Master's spirit, will walk in the steps of His holy and comprehensive love.'[5]

The other formative influence on the style of the Scottish missionary doctor was David Livingstone, one of the first and still the most famous member of this honourable tradition. In 1840, the year before Dr Parker embarked on his tour, Livingstone was appointed by the London Missionary Society to a post in South Africa as a medical missionary, to work as a doctor and a minister.

Livingstone's famous phrase which summed up the forces that he believed would transform Africa and bring it into what he called 'the family of nations' was 'Commerce and Christianity'. This was but a variation of the understanding passionately held by his mentor in South Africa, John Philip, who insisted on the inextricable inter-relatedness of Christianity and Civilisation. His famous dictum summed up Livingstone's belief that the influence of missionary teaching which encompassed the spreading of the Gospel, medical care and education would, when complemented by the opportunity to become involved in world trade through the actions of honest traders, provoke a transformation and uplifting of African life. For this development to take place, however, Africans had to be protected from the depradations of white settlers whose hunger for land had torn apart the traditional societies of South Africa and from the depradations of the Portuguese and Arab slavers. This conclusion was not simply an idea developed in the study, but one produced by his practical knowledge of twelve years working on mission stations in South Africa and the long experience of Dr Philip.

From the outset, Livingstone was clear that as a missionary doctor he had to be committed to constant scientific research and concern. His scientific curiosity never left him. Even in those last dark days when he was desperately ill and near death, his notebook for 1873 still contains careful notes about the fauna and flora of the land through which he was moving so slowly and painfully.

Towards the end of his time in South Africa he was concerned to find a way into the interior where Christianity and Commerce could do their work away from the Boer and British settlers and their greed for land. In his exploratory journeys northward towards the Zambesi basin, he encountered the problems of malaria and tripanosomiasis. He had always kept up his reading of the medical journals which he had arranged to be mailed to him. Now in 1848 he sent for the medical reports on the Niger Expedition of 1841, Dr James McWilliam's *Medical History of the Expedition to the Niger during the Years 1841-2*. He saw that McWilliam's treatment of malaria had not worked all that well but paid particular attention to the careful reports given by the author of the eight autopsies he had performed. As a result of this study and his own observations in the field, Livingstone developed his famous pill made up of quinine and purgatives. On an expedition into malarial territories in 1849 all his patients recovered when dosed by these pills, given in sufficiently large quantities 'to cause ringing in the ears'. He also gave a great deal of thought and investigation to tripanosomiasis but only ventured to try out his ideas about the problem of medication on horses suffering from the equine version of the disease. He did experiment with the use of arsenic with some success. This is one of the early uses of arsenic in a field where it was to be used with some success well into the 20th century.

While still working in the south, he also recorded carefully done surveys of the incidence of a number of diseases common in South Africa, as they occurred in the various areas through which he travelled on his missionary itinerations. He went on to attempt to relate variations in incidence to differences in climate and diet.

In 1853 Livingstone left South Africa for good, committed at first to finding a path for 'Christianity and Commerce' into areas of Africa free from the impact of conflict with white settlers. He later concentrated his efforts on an obsessive and at times frantic attempt to rouse world opinion to bring about international action to end the appalling ravages of the Portuguese and Arab slave raiding in that part of Africa bounded by the Congo in the north and the Zambesi in the south. He retained his medical, scientific and missionary concerns to the end of his life, but he now concentrated on his task as route finder and propagandist.

Clearly, although not trained in the Edinburgh University-EMMS tradition, Livingstone held firmly to their insistence on commitment to rigorous scientific work, as well as to their understanding that medical missionaries were part of the overall task of spreading the Gospel which was to transform the whole human being and human society, not just to save souls. This identity of concern was recognised by the Edinburgh centre when the newly expanded medical and social centre in the Cowgate was named the Livingstone Medical Missionary Training Institution in 1877, four years after Livingstone's death.

Before leaving Livingstone we must take careful note of one area in which his thinking and his practice was radically different from most other missionaries and certainly very different from the majority of whites in Africa throughout most of the 20th century, let alone the 19th. This was his understanding of African traditional medicine. As late as 1951, James McCord (a dedicated medical missionary who had spent his life among the Zulu) could still write that no true Zulu herbalist existed outside the pages of fiction, and that although he did prescribe medicine he was still essentially a smeller-out of witches.[6]

David Livingstone by the mid 1840s had a clear understanding of the belief, fundamental to all the peoples of central and southern Africa, that there was a basic spiritual causation for all disease and that this had to be dealt with along with the symptoms. Without subscribing to their understanding that all evil, and disease is evil, must be caused by the evil intention in someone's heart — either intentionally or subconsciously — he still studied the methods of the nganga or sing'anga. These were essentially healers and in most languages of the Bantu family they are clearly distinguished from the smeller-out of witches (the 'mbisalila' in Chewa/Nyanja, the language best known to this author). He developed great respect for a number of the sing'anga whom he encountered, and began collecting the roots and leaves they used, hoping to create a scientific materia medica. This was one of the projects he gave up when he left South Africa and began the Central African period of his life.

If we look at the formal instructions Livingstone issued to Dr John Kirk, the medical officer of the government-sponsored Zambesi Expedition which he headed in the 1850s, we find a definitive statement of Livingstone's views on African traditional medicine:

> 'One especial means of gaining their favour will be by giving them the benefit of your medical skill and remedial aid. They possess medical men among themselves who are generally the most observant people to be met with; it is desirable to be at all times on good terms with them. In order to this (sic) slight complaints, except among the very poor, ought to be referred to their care, and severe cases, before being undertaken, should be enquired with the doctor himself and no disparaging remark ever made on the previous treatment in the presence of the patient. This line of conduct will lead to the more urgent cases only being referred to you; time and medicine will both be saved, while your influence will be extended.'[7]

This is an attitude in marked contrast to the Edinburgh tradition with which there is otherwise such agreement, indeed identity, of attitude. Rutter Williamson, whose little book is one of the best expositions of this attitude, sees traditional medicine as one of the enemies to be overcome by modern medicine since he lumps all forms of it together as superstition.[8] This attitude stemmed just as much from dogmatic scientism as from dogmatic evangelicalism. Although Livingstone did not have the scientific knowledge of observers of the African scene who continued to decry African traditional medicine into the second half of the 20th century, he was the better scientist. He kept his mind as free as possible from preconceived notions about African medicine, observing and investigating before coming to his very different conclusions.

Neil MacVicar, born in the manse at Manor near Peebles in 1871, is perhaps the man who completely fulfilled the ideals of the movement for medical missionaries in Scotland. He had a deep and indeed passionate faith in God, though he did get into trouble at times because of some disagreement with formal orthodoxy. He was also a brilliant student at Edinburgh University. Like so many other students in the Scottish universities in the 19th century he was poor and got through his course spending five shillings a week for lodgings he could not afford to heat, and five shillings a week for food. For all this he gained several class medals during his course and finally graduated as best student in the graduating class of 1893. He more than fulfilled the insistence of John Lowe, the Director of the EMMS, that any medical missionary had to be a devout person, someone who could deal with harsh conditions and be above the average academically as a medical student.[9]

MacVicar's first appointment was in 1895 to the Blantyre Mission of the Church of Scotland in southern Malawi (then Nyasaland). There he immediately began planning a comprehensive health service for the area influenced by the mission. This was to be based on a central hospital in Blantyre, linked to a series of rural dispensaries which would be run by African 'medical assistants' trained in the central hospital. Even as he began work, with only a makeshift hospital, he initiated the training of these men. When he left Blantyre a few years later one of these trainees, John Gray Kufa, was just setting out for a group of villages across the border in Mozambique where for several years he led a Christian congregation and supervised three 'bush' schools as well as running an extraordinarily busy dispensary on the lines envisaged by MacVicar.[10] This pattern of 'hospital assistant' remained a permanent feature of the Scottish missions in Malawi and was taken up later by the colonial government. (The present writer is most grateful for the skill and care of one such individual and his little hospital in the village where he lived for three years in the 1960s). MacVicar's *Lectures to Hospital Assistants* was published by the Mission Press in 1899 and was much used by others throughout Malawi for many years.

In 1899, it was MacVicar and his medical assistants who ran a massive campaign to check the threat of the invasion of a new strain of smallpox coming into southern Malawi from Mozambique. The colonial authorities expressed their support but could not even provide the lymph necessary for his campaign of vaccination. MacVicar obtained it, through the missions' network, from the Cape Colony. The key to the success of his campaign was the trust he and his assistants had built up among the people so that they received maximum co-operation from the chiefs and elders and, perhaps most important of all in a matrilineal society, the old women of the villages.

At the end of his first tour of duty with the Church of Scotland he was not re-appointed. This was due to misunderstandings and an unimaginative missionary bureaucracy in Edinburgh. A full study of these events can be found in RHW Shepherd, *A South African Medical Pioneer*.

However, on ship while returning to Scotland, MacVicar had met Dr James Stewart, the medical missionary and educationalist who was

Principal of the Lovedale Institution in the then Cape Colony. Stewart had never yet been able to begin effective medical work and training on any permanent basis at Lovedale. When he heard that MacVicar was free he asked him to come to Lovedale and persuaded the authorities of the Free Church of Scotland Mission to accept MacVicar as a medical missionary. In 1902 he arrived at the Cape and supervised the re-opening of the Victoria Hospital which Stewart had built and opened in 1898 only to see it closed during the South African War. The kind of situation that MacVicar was facing can be gauged by the response Stewart had received when he first approached the Department of Internal Affairs of the Cape administration for a subsidy to aid the building of the hospital. The official refused to consider the issue with a curt 'I do not approve of hospitals for Kaffirs'.[11] Luckily Stewart's connections with leading men in the Cape meant that Prime Minister Spriggs was then approached and a subsidy was forthcoming. This helped Stewart to build the Victoria Hospital at Lovedale, the first properly organised and equipped hospital for Africans in the territories that were in 1910 to become the Union of South Africa.

Initially MacVicar thought of developing another medical assistant programme as in Malawi. However, he soon discovered that in the social and political situation of the South African provinces there was not the same role for them to play. Indeed, it was clear that the existing and comparatively well organised health system for whites dominated the medical world and his medical assistants would not be recognised for what they were, something close to what today are often referred to as 'bare-foot doctors'. In this new situation he came to the conclusion that there were three avenues along which medical work should develop for Africans. The first was the training of African nurses. In 1903 he began, with the help of two Scottish missionary nursing sisters, the training of African girls to be nurses and to qualify through the same examination procedures as white nurses. One of the first problems he encountered was in the ward that the Victoria Hospital had for European patients. There he found his nurses were not being treated with the respect that was their due. He therefore persuaded the governing body to close down the European ward rather than have them so abused. The next problem was to get anyone, apart from other missionary bodies, to employ them. Patiently, and with the help of his ministerial colleagues, he persuaded provincial councils, municipal authorities and mining companies to employ them in the clinics these institutions were beginning to provide, albeit to a very inadequate level, for Africans. It is a strange reflection on South African society that as late as 1935, on the eve of MacVicar's retirement, he went as a missionary representative to the Union of South Africa Government Commission on the health care of Africans. There he found, to his astonishment and distress, that the representatives of the Transvaal, the Free State and Natal did not know of the existence of properly qualified African nurses and were ready to oppose any attempt to initiate such training as impossible because of the inadequate intelligence and character of African women. One of these representatives was a distinguished government doctor, the General Superintendent of Johannesburg General Hospital, the biggest in South Africa. MacVicar was able to enlighten his distinguished colleagues as to the existence of a corps of fully trained and formally qualified African nurses already working throughout the Union in mine compound, mission and location clinics which clearly had gained little notice from the leaders of the medical profession. MacVicar's work on that Commission helped to change that situation throughout South Africa and marked the foundations of a nursing profession open to Africans throughout the Union.

His second line of attack on the health problems facing African people in the Union was to develop proper public health studies. No such work had been done at that time with regard to the African population. There are two very famous studies which he undertook in the midst of a crushing schedule of work. The first concerned scurvy. As industry picked up again after the South African War, scurvy reached almost epidemic proportions among the African miners who worked in the mines on the Rand. MacVicar first of all reported accurately on the sheer size of the problem. He then pinned the cause down to the diet provided for the miners in the mine compounds. Until this time the few doctors who had commented on the situation had insisted that the scurvy came from the wet conditions in which the men worked. His final report, published in *The South African Medical Record* of 21 April 1906, led to immediate pressure on the mine companies to change the food provided in the compounds, which, to be fair to them, they did with alacrity. In later years MacVicar also wrote some penetrating analyses on the problem of scurvy in the rural population, whose ability to provide an adequate diet was constantly vulnerable to comparatively minor climatic changes and the impact these had on their crops.

His most famous study was that which he did with the help of missionaries throughout South Africa. This investigated the extent of tuberculosis in the African population. He was able to show that it was spreading rapidly even in what should have been healthy areas like the warm dry northern Cape and on the High Veld. He then went on to show that bovine tuberculosis was not the cause, that in fact the disease had been brought by Europeans to South Africa, a subsidiary source being the Indian community brought by the British into Natal. The disease found a marvellous breeding ground because of the nature of traditional African houses in which everyone slept close together in an essentially badly ventilated space. In addition, pulmonary tuberculosis was making enormous inroads among the mineworkers as a result of the working and living conditions in the mines, and was then being spread into the rural areas by the returning migrant workers. He published his findings in a number of articles before incorporating them in a single study for which Edinburgh University awarded him the MD in 1907. In 1908 this seminal study, still valuable reading today, was published as *Tuberculosis among the South African Natives*.

The third element in his work was the creation of a massive public health campaign among African people within the Union and beyond. He began by initiating health classes for all the students that passed through the Lovedale Institution, at whatever level. This in itself helped to spread a better understanding of diet and hygiene in the rapidly changing African society of South Africa. Old Lovedale pupils then began 'The South African Health Society' which came to have branches throughout the Union and the High Commission Territories. This reliance on African initiative and the devolution of responsibility, a pattern MacVicar began in Malawai, paid off in the rapid growth of this Society. Through the Society, thousands of pamphlets giving basic information about health, hygiene and diet were spread throughout southern Africa. These pamphlets, prepared by MacVicar, were distributed in six languages, including Afrikaans which was of great benefit to the poor white population driven off the land and into the cities by the profound economic changes of the time. He also wrote a *Health Reader* in Xhosa which was soon translated into other languages and came to be used throughout the schools of all the churches and missions in South Africa. Then from 1914, for thirty years, MacVicar edited a quarterly magazine called *Health* which had a wide circulation, containing articles in English, Xhosa and Sotho.

Throughout these years he continued to run the Victoria Hospital and to take an active part in the life of the church as a regular preacher. His life was almost a blueprint of the ideals of the Edinburgh Medical Mission Society, and in so many ways he, like Livingstone, Robert Laws and Willie Scott of Malawi, Clive Irvine of Kenya and many others, believed that the role of the missionary doctor was to bring the good news in word and in deed so as to transform society as well as individuals. This is a totally different understanding from those missionary groups that saw medical care as a 'temporal benefit offered as a bribe for spiritual blessing',[12] or from those who saw it as a distraction from 'soul-saving'.

Nevertheless, MacVicar and all the others, except Livingstone, suffered from one blind spot to a greater or lesser degree. This was their understanding of African traditional healing as simply a terrible superstitious burden from which Africans had to be freed in order for their true humanity to flower. Livingstone saw African traditions of health and healing as something to be explored, understood and related to as did David Rufelle Scott, MacVicar's friend and mentor at Blantyre. Sadly, Scott had not been able to communicate this to MacVicar, in so many ways the paragon of Scottish missionary doctors.

The Scottish missionary doctors still present a challenge to medicine. The challenge is in the form of their antagonism to any form of private practice, and their insistence that the Christian way was that of a health service available to all in which even the poorest received the best possible treatment available. Perhaps most relevant today was their insistence that the creation of good health in the community was as much the goal of medicine as the combatting of disease.

The Scottish Enlightenment and Clinical Medicine

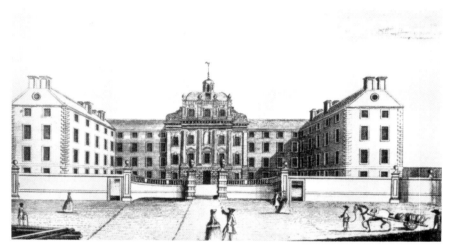

The Royal Infirmary of Edinburgh, 1741-1879, birth-place of Scottish Enlightenment Medicine.

Chapter 8

The Scottish Enlightenment and Clinical Medicine

D Hamilton

Revolution is a grand term, reserved for serious shifts of attitudes. It is a term used of Scottish medicine in two or three periods, the first being the Enlightenment, that period of Scottish dominance in matters cultural and educational in the mid 18th century.[1] The second time of rapid change in which Scotland played such a vital part was the surgical revolution of the mid 19th century which followed but was not part of the Enlightenment. I also suggest that we are just emerging from a period of Scottish dominance in the post-World War II period, dimly perceived, but perhaps clear enough to distinguish it already.

Medicine in the Scottish Enlightenment

From time to time nations become known for their achievement in medical teaching and research. One view is that this is simply the result of a happy coincidence of talented persons in one place; a more exciting explanation is that social factors can explain the emergence and achievement of the group. This dominance means an inevitable decline, and the social forces responsible for the decline can also be sought.[2] The timing of the rise in fame of Scottish medicine is remarkably similar to the dates usually given for the Enlightenment as a whole. The Union of Parliaments in 1707 led to a period of Scottish decline from 1700 roughly to 1720, at which time the economy and confidence in Scotland returned. From 1750-80 was the Golden Age of the cultural Enlightenment. This timing is remarkably similar to the period of growth of the medical school in Edinburgh, as judged by the rising figures for enrolment at the anatomy class.[3] The end of the Enlightenment, in cultural terms, is usually taken as the death of Sir Walter Scott in 1832: this was also the year of the Anatomy Act, made necessary because of the Knox scandal, which showed up the declining medical schools of Scotland in a miserable light.

When describing the medical dimension of the Scottish Enlightenment, commentators often assume that there were remarkable clinical achievements at this time, comparable to the Scottish contributions to philosophy, chemistry, geology, or architecture.[4] In this tranquil century there was cause for medical self-congratulation, and even admiration by later commentators. The great epidemics had gone, and the population was rising. The increasingly self-confident profession saw themselves as at least partly responsible. There is no doubt that some of the Scottish clinicians and anatomists stand out for their scientific work — the Monros *primus* and *secundus*, Robert Whytt, Joseph Black, and Cullen: closer inspection shows that it is for their physiological, anatomical and chemical research that they are known. Whytt's research on the reflex action of the nervous system has eclipsed his considerable efforts to find ways of dissolving bladder stones. Black's renowned work on carbon dioxide has concealed his publication on dyspepsia which accompanied it. Inventions in the bleaching industry and even in water-proofing (what was later called the mackintosh) came from clinicians. In anatomy there were solid achievements, and Monro *secundus* could and did claim to have discovered the lymphatic system. But in clinical medicine no single discovery or lasting innovation stands out, and we look in vain for substantial additions to clinical medicine from these stars of the Enlightenment. Cullen's contribution which was best known to his contemporaries is hardly known today, namely his classification of disease into families and species, along botanical lines, and in this he hardly escaped the ridicule accorded to his contemporary John Brown, whose derivation of a single system of over- and under-stimulation as the explanation for all ills temporarily captured the attention of the medical world. As Gay has concluded, rather harshly, of the medical Enlightenment, 'a tribe of would-be Newtons obstructed progress with their search for a single cause of disease, for a final doctrinaire answer to all questions of health'.[5] Most saw the ills of the body as a disturbance of a self-righting mechanism. Given the right advice and therapy to restore order, disease would be banished.

The medical men of the Enlightenment have been admired for basing their treatment on scientific principles, the basic science of the day. But in physiology at least, this knowledge was deeply flawed. The surgeons can be admired notably for their pragmatic approach to surgical treatment, based on workable methods, and also for their research, which built up a dependable base of anatomical knowledge. But they could be beguiled by faulty theory. Even the surgeons considered the common leg ulcers with which they had to deal as an external manifestation of disordered physiology, and their therapy was appropriate — the creation of another opening on another part of the body to 'let the badness out'. Why then were Scotland and Edinburgh so well-known? Was it simply the success in teaching a new curriculum?

In medical teaching Scotland's claim is that in Edinburgh (followed later by Glasgow and Aberdeen) the Boerhaavian system of teaching students, if not at the bedside then certainly on particular cases, first came to Britain. But this system was and always had been in use for surgical training in the towns of Scotland and on a grand scale in London. The real success in Edinburgh, and later in Scotland as a whole, was that this system was extended to other branches of medicine, especially by the physicians, and as many students as cared to attend were taught. In London the few wealthy physicians made the entry to their rarified specialty as difficult as possible, limiting their student attachments to one or none. In Edinburgh the pedagogical revolution was that a group of teachers agreed to co-operate, giving joint courses of instruction timed to allow students (and the many established doctors who found their way back to Edinburgh for further tuition) to attend a variety of lecture courses. The surgeons in Edinburgh can be admired for their talents for research and in raising their status to be part of university teaching. This they did by means of careful political activity via the Town Council. In turn the Edinburgh physicians can be admired for co-operating with the surgeons, and those teaching midwifery. The lack of power given in the Physicians' Charter left them relatively powerless in Edinburgh.

The result was a town famous for its medical teaching, and the product, a general practitioner, was of immense value to the armed forces of the day, and indeed to any community outside the larger towns. The training in midwifery, though controversial, also met the new needs of the day. In this response we see the role of Adam Smith's views and the assumptions that teaching responds to the market forces, giving a demand-led medical curriculum rather than a teacher-dominated one, as in London.[6] This rapprochement may have been the product of a group loss of confidence in Edinburgh after the Union. Certainly the town looked actively for new ventures, and the old craft divisions in medicine could not be sustained in this new pragmatism. Just as the physicians were prepared to accept surgeons as equals, so the objections to manual work by the learned had also gone. Anatomical work and painting was encouraged. The *literati* of Edinburgh were also prepared to deal directly with printers, manufacturers and industrialists. There were, however, limits — a physician and even a senior surgeon would not wish to conduct or be seen at an autopsy; instead, a report would be brought to him.

The Infirmary
The second feature of Enlightenment medicine is also less obvious. The rise of the hospital, notably Edinburgh's Royal Infirmary, reveals that the consumers, namely the ordinary citizens, were for the first time generally agreed that orthodox medicine not only had something to offer, but that it offered more than the alternative sources of healing — notably the local folk healers, wise women, healing wells and so on. When looking at the therapy given in the Edinburgh Royal Infirmary by the physicians, devoted almost entirely to purging, induced vomiting and other evacuant therapy, it is remarkable that the patients should regard the therapy so highly, but it seems that this was so. Patients stayed in the hospital for months on end: few fled the wards, and most came out alive.[7] Part of this establishment of orthodoxy, which can be admired in Edinburgh, was the simplification of the pharmacopoeia. In spite of the remaining complexity of therapy, there was a new pragmatism and nihilism about older therapies, many of which were being culled from the textbooks. The influence of David Hume and the other Scottish philosophers is seen in this: the retreat from groundless speculation and the reliance on the evidence of the senses in receiving information on the world must have influenced day-to-day clinical life. Hume's views that the senses could distort the evidence as it accumulated must have made the clinicians wary of extravagant claims for novelties. This sceptical shift also meant the rejection of passive acceptance of the view that God's hidden plans had to be accepted: instead man's body was increasingly placed in secular care. There was, in this atmosphere, less fear of the afterlife, and indeed some doubt that there was one. No-one would contemplate death without an attempt at medication first, and this shift from care of the soul to study and attendance on the body perhaps was not unrelated to the importance of anatomy and painting in the Enlightenment. But above all there was hope of progress: the

student petition summoning Cullen from Glasgow to Edinburgh spoke of his 'ardour for improvement and spirit of liberal enquiry in medicine'.

In the Infirmary there was, for the first time, the opportunity to observe quite large groups of patients. By mid-century the crowded Royal Infirmary of Edinburgh could accommodate up to 228 patients and gave opportunities for observation and experience which were quite new. Prior to the appearance of the Infirmary, the physician or surgeon, in Edinburgh and elsewhere, earned his living from entrepreneurial private practice, or teaching. For the physician these patients were few, scattered and paid well. Moreover, a physician like Cullen might ethically prescibe by post. Follow-up was also rare, and the evolution of disease was accordingly poorly understood. In a hospital, however, the patients were numerous and the death rate was low. Those chosen to teach the students had amplified their patient numbers and the simplification of the pharmacopoeia may have had its roots in the rise of the hospital.

Physicians like Cullen and Gregory may have been forced to admit that with their mass experience of treatment, using the less expensive remedies available in the Infirmary for the poor, their grand schemes of therapy suitable for the rich (the exotic diets and expensive regimen of holidays and so forth) proved no better nor worse than the economical therapies available in hospital. Moreover, Cullen attempted to simplify therapy, preferring to lose a patient to illness rather than kill by the therapy.

But follow-up of the patient was poor even for the hospital patient. It is interesting that those Scottish men entering military service, like James Lind, John Pringle and Gilbert Blane, had more opportunity to follow up disease than had their teachers, and the doctors in the armed forces could innovate in a way denied others by watching the numerous ill persons confined to ships and barracks' hospitals or the like.[8] They were also accustomed to making statistical returns on the incidence of disease. It may even be that post-mortem opportunities were greater in the forces. By the end of the century, observation of groups of patients, experiments with new drugs and an experimental approach characterised the Scottish scene. Earlier, the esteemed journal *Medical Observations and Essays*, first published in 1731, said that it reserved the right to reject essays deficient in facts. A little-known book by Gilbert Blane, his *Medical Logic* of 1819, perhaps sums up the Scottish approach, one which may have pervaded the teaching he received. Blane referred to 'the absurd positions of Pitcairn, the puerile and shallow hypotheses of Boerhaave and Sylvius'. He then advocated an alternative: 'If the benefits derivable from physiological science are so limited, from what other and better source is improvement to come? The answer is from accurate observation; in other words enlightened empiricism'.

When and why did this Scottish dominance end? Firstly, the numerical dominance in teaching continued into the 19th century, but the old flair had gone, and the medical schools in Edinburgh and Glasgow were notable for petty internal feuds and pamphleteering. Moreover, England had opened medical schools on the Scottish model. First France then Germany dominated medical development, based on a new physiology from experimentation. Scotland was shackled. Though some experimental physiology was carried out, there was growing hostility to vivisection among those in authority and growing resistance to the idea of autopsy after death. The lack of bodies for dissection after death culminated in the Burke and Hare scandal which set a serious barrier against dissection in general, and post-mortem in particular, in Scotland and Britain. Even the fact that the Anatomy Act was drawn up in London, and showed a lack of familiarity with Scottish law, reflects on the decline in Scotland. Scottish medicine was seen as unprincipled and squalid, where expedience rather than morality was important. Furthermore, the doctors were becoming richer, and less dependent on teaching, and perhaps less keen on research. American medical students opted for Paris instead of Edinburgh. Of the famous Paris medical teachers one student wrote home: 'here chariots and guineas are not the aim'.

The great 19th century Scottish contributions are outside the period of the Enlightenment and quite distinct from it. Simpson's discovery of chloroform was a major extension of a general approach to anaesthesia pioneered elsewhere. Lister's contributions are those of a solitary entrepreneur with few if any roots in the now creaking Scottish system, a system which was sluggish compared to the vitality of Continental research and teaching. In Scotland the petty quarrels and litigation continued. Even Simpson denigrated Lister, and such feuds contrast with the harmony of the 18th century. Simpson can be seen as one of the new breed of Continental experimenters, but Lister fits awkwardly into any attempt to see these men as part of a Scottish tradition. If there was a local factor, then it was that in Glasgow Lister came face to face with the massive problem of the growing death-rate in hospitals and in particular after surgery. Because of Glasgow's size and the evils of the Industrial Revolution, Lister turned his efforts to understanding and dealing with the problem. It was a slow revolution in surgery, partly because of the ineffectiveness of carbolic acid dressings at the start.

The last period I wish to discuss briefly is that of the decades immediately post-World War II, a period which has curious similarities to the events in the 18th century. Scotland continued to produce large numbers of medical graduates, but the feature was the export of large numbers of trained staff, notably academics and surgeons. In this matter, Glasgow followed and perhaps outshone Edinburgh, though it is a trend that can be followed in departments headed by Wilkie through Learmonth to Illingworth. I believe other factors were at work. Firstly the Scottish hospitals were merged into five larger Regional Hospital Boards which not only had the universities at their centre, but also had in each area numerous small hospitals with specialty interests. This enabled teaching of the rapidly growing numbers of clinical specialties, whereas the English hospitals were handicapped by the teaching hospitals' traditional detachment, physically and organisationally, from the surrounding hospitals. Secondly, NHS salaries enabled many to seek a career in research or specialty medicine without need or thought of doing private practice, a dispensation which gave Scotland an advantage over England and must have pervaded the attitudes and assumptions in the medical faculties and schools.

The constant expansion of the NHS came to an end in the 1960s and retrenchment followed: the end of another revolutionary period had been reached.

CHAPTER 9

A Not-so-plain Tale from the Raj

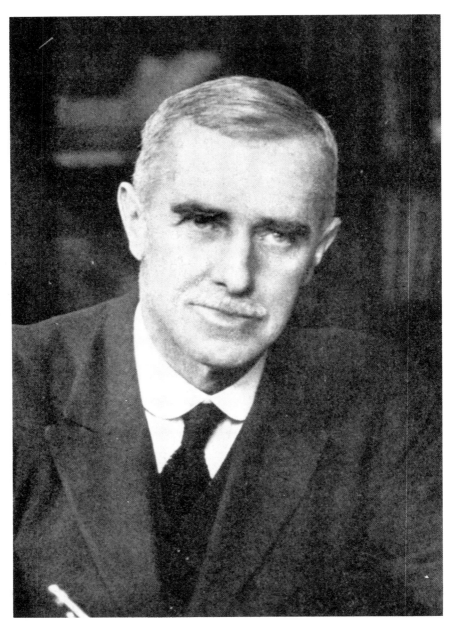

Anderson Gray McKendrick, photographed during his years as Superintendent of the Laboratory of the Royal College of Physicians of Edinburgh.

Chapter 9
A Not-so-plain Tale from the Raj: A G McKendrick, IMS

J Aitchison and G S Watson

Mathematics and Medicine

On 22 April 1829 that august body, the Senatus of the University of Glasgow, forwarded a report from its Medical Faculty to the Royal Commissioners appointed to visit the Universities of Scotland. The Commission was intended to reform both the curriculum and administration of the higher education system, and the medical professors left the Commissioners in no doubt as to their views on the utility of mathematics as a prerequisite for medical education:

> 'It is now generally admitted that no worse set of theorists or more inert and blundering practitioners ever existed than the mathematical Physicians. And that those habits which are requisite for a good medical practitioner are rather injured than improved by a profound knowledge of Mathematics.'

It is perhaps surprising to find the same University happily accepting as Principal from 1907 to 1929 one such mathematical physician, a Cambridge Wrangler no less, Sir Donald MacAlister. Indeed it could be reasonably claimed that he is now more widely remembered for his mathematical invention of 1879, that indispensable tool of many medical statistical investigations, the lognormal distribution.[1] And today we doubt if more than one member of the Senate of that University is aware that it nurtured one of the greatest contributors to our knowledge of the relationship of mathematics and medicine, namely the very remarkable Anderson Gray McKendrick.

Some biographical details

Anderson Gray McKendrick was born in Edinburgh in 1876, the fifth and last of the children of John Gray McKendrick and Mary Souttar. A few months later his father was appointed to the Chair of the

Institutes of Medicine in the University of Glasgow, where he remained until his retirement in 1906. (The Chair was renamed as Physiology in 1893, midway through McKendrick's tenure). Anderson was thus brought up in the heyday of the West End of Glasgow, in the bustling academic household of a vigorous and colourful father, a devoted mother and medical student lodgers,[2] boarded to counteract John Gray's use of his income to purchase necessary experimental equipment, including 'a suitable place for frogs'.[3] By all accounts John Gray had an exceptional flair for experimental physiological research and was a popular lecturer;[4] he revelled, for example, in his Royal Institution Christmas Lectures which contained such conclusions as 'Frogs have been of more service to humanity than all the lions and tigers in the world.'[5] He was a devout Christian combining 'temperance' with a good table, and an obsessive music-lover. Even his retirement was full of tireless activity, with his passion for music motivating his construction of what must be one of the earliest outdoor attempts at hi-fi reproduction.[6]

Next door to the family home in Westbourne Gardens lived George Levack, a widowed merchant with six daughters (at the last count). In such circumstances the emergence of Miss Levack's Establishment for the Education of Young Ladies seemed inevitable. With two elder sisters young Anderson was destined to spend his early schooldays in this embryonic Westbourne School for Girls.[7] With such an educational start to life what boy could fail to make his academic mark? He told his own family in later years that he learned more from the Misses Levack than from any other teachers. Later, at Kelvinside Academy, any flair which he may have displayed seems to have been eclipsed by his prize-winning older brother, John Souttar.

It seemed natural that John Gray's three sons should all study medicine in the University of Glasgow. All three graduated with high commendation,[8] Anderson completing his course in 1900 after what appears to have been a leisurely paced approach and with a year out to study at the University of Jena.

Choice of career in the Indian Medical Service

The subsequent choice of career seems to have been determined by father McKendrick. Willie, the eldest of the family, had died in 1893, a year after graduation, of phthisis in South Africa, the sanatorial Switzerland of that time for British victims of tuberculosis.[9] John Souttar was now established in general practice in Buckingham

Terrace, and there was, in John Gray's thinking at least, no room for two McKendricks in practice in Glasgow. A natural alternative in those days was the Indian Medical Service (IMS); a perusal of the *Glasgow University Magazine (GUM)*, the student newspaper of the day, reveals active recruitment around the British universities with emphasis on the variety of careers in clinical practice and research that it offered.[10] From Glasgow alone we find near contemporaries of McKendrick in the Service: NEH Scott as civil surgeon, J Drummond Graham as medical administrator, WG Liston as research bacteriologist. McKendrick was to create a new form of service.

With choice of career settled, the young graduate took digs in London to study with specialist crammers[11] for the IMS written examination in February 1901. He came first[12] and then, as surgeon on probation, began training in military and tropical medicine at the Army School at Netley, finishing second[13] in the overall London and Netley examinations in June 1901.

An influential meeting with Ronald Ross

Young Lieutenant McKendrick was spared Lord Northbrook's long exhortation[14] at the Netley prize-giving by being sent on special duty to study anti-malarial techniques in Sierra Leone with Ronald Ross on the fifth Liverpool Malarial Expedition.[15] Ross had discovered the final, and Nobel Prize-winning, connection between the Anopheles mosquito and malaria in man while serving in the IMS and had already carried out a number of apparently successful anti-malarial expeditions. Although his new student fully understood, and approved of, Ross's techniques he was never to be allowed to implement them in India, feeling bitterly disappointed when the half-promise of command of an anti-mosquito campaign on the island of Bombay failed to materialise. In a letter to Ross dated 6 August 1911 he wrote:

> 'I have not written you since I left Bombay and the reason was that I was so disgusted, that I just had to keep my "grouse" to myself. It was horribly disappointing, but as it happened it was the best thing that could have happened to me for I found a wife here, and now we have a boy — a splendid fellow of 8 months.'[16]

The expedition, however, proved seminal to the young IMS Lieutenant in a quite different way. By a stroke of good scientific fortune Ross and McKendrick returned home early and together on board the SS *Sobo*,[17] remembered as the SS *Jebba* by McKendrick. Ross was a polymath and a major part of the 'poly' was a substantial

knowledge and ability in mathematics. He had already started on a
rather complex mathematical model describing the various aspects of
the transmission of malaria, which was to be extended later into a
more general theory which he termed *A Priori Pathometry*.[18] We know
from later correspondence that on this voyage he enthused over the
usefulness of mathematical reasoning in the theory and practice of
medicine and that he found an eager listener, indeed a convert, in the
young IMS officer. On 5 October 1901 McKendrick wrote to Ross:

> 'I am writing for the books you advised: and hope to go out well equiped (sic)
> at the end of the month.'[19]

And later, on 24 November 1908, he acknowledged Ross's influence:

> 'You may be interested to hear that I started off on Mathematics a couple of
> years ago, and find it most useful. The calculus is always coming in in work,
> and also probabilities are very useful. That is a late result of your stimulus
> onboard the Jebba.'[20]

Official duties

For new recruits to the IMS there was a prescribed period of military
service before civil duty could be assumed. McKendrick spent eighteen
months in the Somaliland campaigning against the Mahdi, a major
contribution being the construction of a tank of safe water for the
troops, and a minor contribution being a form of pre-ENSA
entertainment of his fellow officers on what must have been a uniquely
portable musical instrument, an ocarina of Dresden china.[21]

On his return to India he was soon posted to civil duties in the
cantonment of Kasauli, in the Himalayan foothills south of Simla.
After much prevarication the Indian Government, cajoled by its IMS
officers and by the *British Medical Journal*,[22] had founded in 1900 its own
Pasteur Institute of India in this hill station. No longer would soldiers
bitten by mad dogs in India have to be sent to Paris for treatment;
even Viceroys were vulnerable.[23] Apart from a short spell as
Government Statistical Officer in Simla, McKendrick's official duties
were to lie in the treatment, including the preparation of vaccine, and
study of rabies[24],[25], not only in Kasauli but also for a shorter period
in the South India Pasteur Institute at Coonoor, near Ooty. Historians
regard him as a distinguished IMS rabies expert of his day[26], and after
retirement from the IMS he added substantially to this reputation by
a series of nine statistical reviews of the results of antirabic treatment
in Pasteur Institutes throughout the world (conducted on behalf of the

Health Section of the League of Nations), and by thirty-eight critical reviews of the rabies literature in the *Tropical Diseases Bulletin*.

Most men would have settled for such a full, satisfactory and satisfying career. McKendrick had, however, inherited his father's restless urge for research, had listened as a young man to the many academic visitors to the McKendrick good table such as Lord Kelvin, Sir James Dewar and Sir William Ramsay[27]; above all, he had been transformed by his personal catalyst, Ronald Ross.

Interlude

No sensitive young doctor working in India in the first decade of this century could remain unaffected by the prevalence of epidemic and endemic diseases such as malaria, cholera, plague, typhoid, kala-azar and the millions of lives these claimed each year. After some self-study in mathematics culminating in a paper on serum dynamics[28] — critical of Ehrlich and Arrhenius, acclaimed by Donnan and Ross[29] and later developed by Zinsser[30] — he set towards a study of how mathematical models might be used to describe epidemiological phenomena with a view to their use as tools for the formulation of practical policies of control. Mellor's *Higher Mathematics*[31] must have been his mathematical bible.[32] It is an ideal text on mathematics and its non-trivial application; it would serve well today as corrective reading for school boys and girls inculcated with the abstraction of the 'new mathematics'.

The successful application of mathematics to real problems requires in the applier a fine judgement between the degree of simplicity which will allow tractable mathematical development and the apparently complex structure of the problem. In all his subsequent work McKendrick had this judgement in abundance; he was in our view a natural applied mathematician. It is, of course, difficult to substantiate such a claim for a largely non-mathematical audience. But let us try with one of the earliest and simplest examples of his genius.

The great opsonic index controversy

In the early years of this century there occurred an episode of medical history which may be termed the *great opsonic index controversy*, involving three prominent figures as principals: Sir Almroth Wright, McKendrick's Professor of Pathology at Netley and by this time at St Mary's Hospital; Karl Pearson, a founding grandfather of modern statistics at the biometric laboratory at University College London; and George

Bernard Shaw, critic and playwright. It was a complex affair and we shall concentrate on the essential points as they involve our story. Shaw in his play *The Doctor's Dilemma*, particularly in its Preface, gives a good account of the argument; for Ridgeon read Wright.

Central to any resolution of the controversy must be the ability of the pathologist to measure accurately the degree of phagocytosis activity of the leucocytes of an infected person. The total number of bacteria gobbled up by 100 leucocytes from a blood sample of the infected person was determined by microscopic inspection, and this was divided by the total number in 100 leucocytes from a normal person. This ratio was the *opsonic index*, an early and crude form of assay or calibration which was even celebrated in a student song of the day.[33] To judge the reliability of such an index clearly requires an ability to describe the pattern of variability of bacteria counts over individual leucocytes, such as in the following Table.

													Totals
Number of leucocytes	12	16	22	17	11	6	5	3	3	2	1	1	1	100
Number of contained bacteria	0	1	2	3	4	5	6	7	8	9	10	11	12	311

This problem attracted the attention of Karl Pearson and his followers at University College London. Pearson had already developed his complicated system of curves to describe patterns of variability in *continuous* measurement and these were applied mercilessly to every bacterial count data set in sight.[34] This Pearsonian approach was doomed to failure. Apart from the absurdity of attempting to describe so obviously discrete variability by a continuous pattern, the many parameters required in a fitted form such as are virtually uninterpretable. It is an excellent example of a familiar statistical ailment known as concentrating on goodness of model fit at the expense of simplicity.

Pearson at this time was at loggerheads with Wright over the nature of scientific method. Pearson was advocating early forms of controlled trials whereas Wright was an experientialist,[35] arguing that the human mind learns from experience in a complex, unanalysable way. WF Harvey, IMS pathologist, Director of the Indian Central Research Institute at Kasauli and a life-long colleague and friend of McKendrick, was so disturbed by this dispute between his Netley professor and Pearson that he took study leave in 1909, spending his mornings with Pearson at UCL and his afternoons and evenings with Wright at St. Mary's.[36] The outcome was a joint paper[37] on the opsonic index by Harvey and McKendrick, written by Harvey and incorporating an unpublished study by McKendrick. It is interesting for its long discussion of the relationship of the statistician to the clinician but it had not yet escaped from the Pearsonian system of curves.

By 1912 McKendrick had made the major breakthrough,[38] astonishing in its simplicity. A leucocyte starts life empty of bacteria. It may go on and capture one bacterium, then possibly another to make a total of two, and so on. Phagocytosis is a process in time and we should start by considering how changes take place in a single leucocyte. In the diagram time flows left to right.

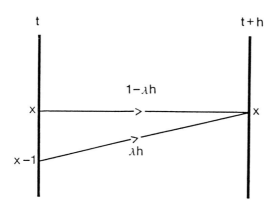

Consider a *short* interval from time t to t+h. How can we arrive at x bacteria in our leucocyte at time t+h? Only in two ways.

1) There are x—1 bacteria at time t and our leucocyte eats another bacterium in the short interval h.

2) There are already x bacteria at time t and our leucocyte fails to eat another bacterium in the short time interval.

If we postulate that the probability of a bacterium catch is proportional to the time interval considered we can then write the probability of a move from x—1 at t to x at t+h as λ h and the probability of no move from x at t to x at t+h as $1 - \lambda$ h. If $P_x(t)$ denotes the probability of there being x bacteria in a leucocyte at time t then the simple grammar of the language of probability demands the following relationship:

$$P_x(t+h) = \lambda\, hp_{x-1}(t) + (1-\lambda h)p_x(t).$$

Rearrangement and narrowing of the interval h produces what is now termed a differential-difference equation

$$\frac{dp_x(t)}{dt} = \lambda\{P_{x-1}(t) - P_x(t)\}$$

from which an explicit form

$$P_x(t) = \frac{e^{-\lambda t}(\lambda t)^x}{x!}$$

emerges. Note that, in contrast to the Pearsonian approach, this pattern of variability involves only one parameter λ, interpretable as the rate of phagocytosis, and McKendrick had no difficulty in showing excellent goodness-of-fit to opsonic data. The work[39] was published in *Science Progress* of which Ross was editor.

This *tour de force* from someone with no formal mathematical training and working in the isolation of Indian hill-stations is truly remarkable. Necessity is certainly the mother of invention: possibly isolation is the father of genius.

The formal mathematics described above and now known as the Poisson process leading to the Poisson distribution had been developed some years earlier but this in no way detracts from this particular achievement of McKendrick. It is clear that he was unaware of this previous work.[40] Interestingly this same paper goes further and gives undoubtedly the first development of what is now known as the homogeneous birth process, usually ascribed to a slightly later paper,[41] itself described as 'remarkably early'.[42]

Two years previously Captain McKendrick, as he now was, had read an equally fundamental paper at an Indian Malarial Congress. This appeared[43] in 1912 in a short-lived Indian journal entitled *Paludism*, which was a pilot for the *Indian Journal of Medical Research*. The modelling of epidemic processes by differential equations was similar to that described above with different transition rates allowing the description of a variety of epidemic types: itch in guinea pigs (a single population problem); syphilis (a two population male-and-female problem; malaria (a host and vector problem).

McKendrick's views on mathematics and medicine

By all accounts McKendrick was a kind, modest, even retiring, Christian gentleman. He would certainly have strongly disapproved of this weekend conference and, in particular, the timing of this lecture to coincide with Presbyterian sermons. Only in matters relating to mathematically-oriented research does he seem to have expressed passionate views. In his letter of 5 December 1912 to Ross about his opsonic index work he wrote:

> 'The Pearsonians have as usual made a frightful hash of the whole business. That may sound a strong argument, but the only hope for statistical work is a priori reasoning, and K. Pearson has raised an opposition by ill-advised methods, and ill applied results, which will take years to overcome . . .. I do not know whether you favour Pearsonian methods, but I must earnestly hope you do not. In the differential equations of epidemic action we have the true starting point, and it is from these that we should start. ... I have just come back from the Sanitary and Malaria Conference in Madras. The work was terrific, though the proceedings may read tamely. The malaria procs. were so, because I had a battle royal with Bentley, who had twisted our mathl. reasoning beyond understanding, and beyond reason. The fight lasted 8 hours, but in the end he withdrew a paper, which would have upset our whole programme, and covered us with disgrace if it had been passed, and accepted. He is a strange chap. If he wanted to go from London to Paris, he would prefer to go via Tokyo, and then he would advertise a new route. To keep these men on the rails is the bane of my life.'[44]

In 1913 there came at last with study leave the opportunity of formal training in mathematics:

> 'I am coming home in March for a 2 years spell. Mostly for study, and I am going to settle rigidly down to Mathematics if I can get the powers to agree. As you know I am self taught, and with 2 years leave, I wish to get myself thoroughly grounded. Will you be in London in March? I would like to see you. We shall be passing through enroute for Stonehaven, where I shall spend most of my time. I shall work in Aberdeen. Gilbert Walker (Boomerang Walker, F.R.S. who is chief of observatories here) has helped me no end: and above all he has shown me the advantage of a rigidness which is at present beyond me, and which seems to be only attainable by study in the regular channels.'[45]

There is no time here to detail the flow of papers which emerged from this stimulus.

Work in Edinburgh

There is no evidence that a letter[46] dated 26 June 1919 to the *Indian Medical Gazette* seeking a mathematical fellow-spirit in the IMS brought any response. Subsequent events would have indeed made such collaboration difficult since soon afterwards McKendrick developed that scourge of the hill stations, tropical sprue or hill diarrhoea, with repeated long and debilitating recurrences over the next ten years. He retired on medical grounds from the IMS with the rank of Lieutenant-Colonel in 1920, settling in Edinburgh with his wife and four young children. There he was soon to be appointed Superintendent of the Research Laboratory of the Royal College of Physicians of Edinburgh[47] where he remained until his retirement in 1941. These were tough days for the McKendrick family with little money, Indian-reared children susceptible to Western infections, a sick though resilient father and an inexperienced maid who, by destroying the visiting cards of Edinburgh ladies, delayed by a number of years the acceptance of the family into Edinburgh society.

Despite all these misfortunes and the heavy administrative load which the routine laboratory analysis of specimens and research programme involved, the fire to apply mathematics was unquenched. In this brief account of McKendrick's work in mathematical and statistical modelling it is possible only to touch on two of the many developments. Befriended and encouraged by Sir Edmund Whittaker, Professor of Mathematics in the University of Edinburgh, McKendrick continued the development of his epidemic theory by reading a penetrating and wide-ranging paper[48] on 'Applications of Mathematics to Medical Problems' to the Edinburgh Mathematical Society in 1926. This paper has subsequently been so highly thought of that it was republished and analysed in great detail by Dr JO Irwin in his Presidential Address[49] to the Royal Statistical Society in 1962; it is also reprinted in Conolly and Oliveria-Pinto's book[50] on 'Selected Papers in Applicable Mathematics' as their best example of the relevance of mathematics to medicine.

The second development over the years 1927-39 was a series of five 'Contributions to the Mathematical Theory of Epidemics'[51] from a deterministic approach in collaboration with WO Kermack. Kermack was a young biochemist at the Research Laboratory, already totally blinded by a caustic soda explosion while working alone one evening in the laboratory.[52] An important aspect of these papers, now repeatedly referred to by researchers who have seldom read them, is the 'threshold theorem': the introduction of infectious cases into a community of susceptibles does not give rise to an epidemic outbreak if the density of susceptibles is below a critical value. If, however, the critical value is exceeded, there is an epidemic of magnitude sufficient to reduce the density of susceptibles as far below the threshold as it originally was above. Such a result, clearly important in the quantitative way in which it relates the threshold to the rate of infectivity, is now quoted in almost every paper on epidemic theory, and interestingly in one on the spatial spread of diseases such as rabies,[53] the disease of McKendrick's official duties. There can be little doubt that we shall soon see it referenced in a paper on AIDS.

There were fun papers too, not least the concept of an infinite Mobius strip,[54] colourfully reported in *The Scotsman* the morning after its presentation to the Edinburgh Mathematical Society by the blind Kermack.[55]

Disappointments

According to his obituary writer, WF Harvey:

> 'McKendrick realised full well that much of his research presented a closed book to his fellow-medicals who were seldom equipped in mathematical analysis.'[56]

There was in the early days a substantial resistance to the introduction of random processes into the description of physiological and pathogenic processes within the human body. McKendrick was well aware of this; although his choice of title *The Physical Aspect of the Opsonic Experiment* asserts his belief in the mathematical modelling he is at pains to persuade the resistant reader:

> 'It may be argued, however, that no comparison can be drawn between the conduct of a molecule of a gas and that of a living cell; that whilst, where there is no life, particles may follow random paths, such will not be the case with living cells which are apparently capable of voluntary movement and effort. (Such movements are no doubt chemio-tactic and only simulate voluntary movements.) But on the other hand it must be remembered that the leucocyte is in an environment of particles of food of an equally tempting nature which are scattered at random in its vicinity. It need only browse at random as a cow browses over a fat pasture.'

He must have felt particularly piqued by the poohpoohing remarks in the discussion of his paper on 'House infection in cholera and cancer'[57] by Professor Russell who, according to a *British Medical Journal* report, 'pointed out that statistics were often misleading and the law of averages open to grave misinterpretation.'[58] We know the feeling well. Even today we have experience of addressing a medical audience on the role of the statistician in medicine, in particular in statistical diagnosis, emphasising that the statistician's interest and particular expertise is in the handling of uncertainty and variability. If the *BMJ* reporter had been there he could have recorded that in the discussion 'Professor X pointed out that patients were much too variable for statistics to be applied successfully to them'. There is no accounting for the variability of defence mechanisms.

There is little doubt that McKendrick was bitterly disappointed that his pioneering work in mathematical epidemiology went virtually unrecognised during his lifetime:

> 'A man's reach must exceed his grasp. And I suppose that every young scientist attempts more than he can tackle, and hopes to see himself in the Royal in the distant future.'[59]

Whittaker, we understand, had no doubt that McKendrick should have attained Fellowship of the Royal Society. There was some hitch in his nomination and, of course, such processes of distinction are still clouded in secrecy and mystery. In retrospect there can be little doubt that McKendrick was far ahead of his time and may have suffered from a view that other than physical applications of mathematics were not quite respectable.

Recognition

It is sad, though not in the least surprising, that recognition came soon after his death in 1943 and his research papers are widely quoted today: a quick glance at the *Science Citation Index* will confirm this. His work is now universally acclaimed throughout the community of researchers in mathematical epidemiology and stochastic processes. Early discoverers of his work were DG Kendall,[60] MS Bartlett[61] and JO Irwin[62]. Whole papers have been devoted to aspects of his work:[63] the latest to come our way is a critique of how his work on population biology has influenced mathematics.[64] To the earnest biographer who has trained himself to spot the name McKendrick at fifty paces, imagine the breakfast surprise and delight to unfold Hong Kong's quality newspaper, the *South China Morning Post*, and spot an unsolicited reference.[65]

There is a delightful, affectionate and very well informed Christmas card sent to the McKendrick family in 1918 — probably by Pasteur Institute clients. It seems to sum up the whole story, and must have been a source of great joy to McKendrick. A few verses gave the flavour of the man and his hobby.

A

Kasauli Doggerel

to

Major A.G. McKendrick

McKendrick, he's a doctor,
And lives Kasauli way.
He spends much time in stabbing,
"Little Marys" every day.

He's tall, and very courtly,
His smile, and looks are warm.
His hobby, sounding awesome,
Need cause you no alarm.

Though classed as Mathematics,
Its name is like a word
Resembling "Osculation",
Of which, of course, you've heard.

But Oscillating Variants
Are quite another thing,
Though they, too, solve a problem
Of how infections spring.

Just "why" and "when" and "wherefore"
We mortals should succumb
To bites of dogs called rabid,
Or lickings of their tongue.

So, to our braw McKendrick,
His wife, and bairnies four,
We wish a Happy Christmas,
Love, Health, and Luck galore.

Medicine as a true mathematical science

By themselves, mathematical models of epidemic and other medical
processes can achieve nothing. Eradication of epidemic diseases clearly
depends on the existence of clinical means, of reducing the infectivity
of human beings (vaccination, inoculation) and of reducing sources of
infection (isolation, spraying of mosquito breeding grounds, etc). It
also requires economic, political and manpower resources to implement
any selected plan. What mathematical epidemic models can and do
supply is a non-experimental means of assessing the effectiveness of

alternative plans and indeed of determining an optimum policy. For our advanced knowledge of these we are in McKendrick's debt.

Whatever our views may be on that 1829 minute of the Glasgow Senate, or more generally on the relation of mathematics and statistics to medicine, Ronald Ross and Anderson Gray McKendrick were in no doubt. Ross wrote to McKendrick in 1911:

> 'I believe that you and I are the only persons living who have touched the subject as yet and I think that you should be allowed to work it out, even if I can do no more at it. If they give you an assistant later on, it will suffice and I will get one for you. But let us first block out the big masses of malariometry and pathometry in general. Let me know however if this idea meets with general approval, as I think it will. . . . We shall end by establishing a new science. But first let you and me unlock the door and then anybody can go in who likes.'[66]

A year later McKendrick wrote to Ross:

> 'The time will come I am sure when your name will be associated with the reduction of Medicine to a true mathematical science, even more than with the discovery of the mosquito carrier. That seems a far cry at present, but there is some thing grand and big in the laws which emerge, and they are fundamental. I hope some day soon you may bring out a book on Mathematics and Medicine, and I hope I shall be able to contribute a chapter.'[67]

It could be argued that McKendrick should have written the book with a chapter by Ross.

Acknowledgements
We are delighted that two of McKendrick's 'bairnies four', Joyce and Margot, now Mrs Joyce Matthew and Mrs Stuart McWilliam, were able to attend the Congress with other members of the Clan McKendrick. We would like to express our gratitude to the family and to countless others for all their help in our study of the life and work of Anderson Gray McKendrick. Professor Watson also gratefully acknowledges support from the National Science Foundation, Grant MCS 842-1301.

CHAPTER 10

Scotland and Australasia

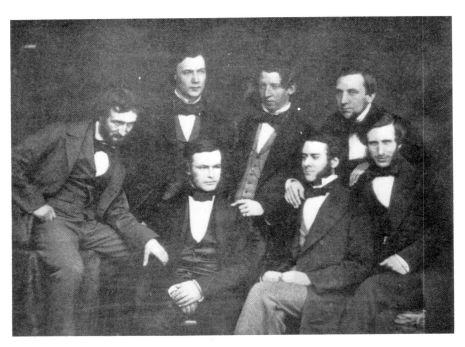

The Residents, Royal Infirmary of Edinburgh, 1854. George Hogarth Pringle, in the checked waistcoat, is standing with his left hand resting on Joseph Lister's shoulder.

Chapter 10
Scotland and Australasia
D A Dow

In a recent article the Australian historian Eric Richards identified fifteen specific groups of immigrants to Australia from Scotland — 'convicts, governors, merchants, administrators, labourers, capitalists, domestic servants, pastoral pioneers, artists, writers, doctors, educators, miners, men of religion, drovers' wives, and many others'.[1] Both in this instance, and in a subsequent article on Scottish emigration[2], Richards paid scant attention to doctors as a specific group, although he acknowledged that the Scots were prominent among the medical practitioners of Colonial Australia.[3] Since this assessment was based on his examination of the first two volumes of the *Australian Dictionary of Biography* it is neither comprehensive nor, more critically, representative.

The evident limitations in Richards' comments are indicative of the paucity of research into the influence of Scottish medicine on Australasia. This paper will attempt to identify some of the major themes awaiting illumination.

The 1988 Australian Bicentennial celebrations will undoubtedly focus attention on many aspects of that country's history and, in particular, its relationship with the United Kingdom from the time the First Fleet sailed for Botany Bay in the autumn of 1787. It is questionable, however, if medicine will feature prominently in these studies, despite its central importance to the well-being and growth of the new settlements which emerged in the 19th century. With a glorious disregard for chronology, the Irish-Australian historical community have already celebrated the Bicentenary, at a conference held in 1983. The resulting volume of proceedings, edited by Colm Kiernan and entitled *Australia and Ireland 1788-1988. Bicentenary Essays*, was subsequently published in 1986.[4] Of the twenty-five essays included in Kiernan's volume, two were devoted exclusively to studies of Irish emigration to Australia. Between them, the two authors made only one fleeting reference to medicine, as one of the two meritocratic professions (along with engineering) where Irishmen gained approximately their due proportion of appointments.[5] No statistics were provided to substantiate this claim, and none of the other twenty-three contributors raised the subject of health care.

Numerically far greater than their Irish counterparts, the Scottish doctors in Australasia have fared little better at the hands of scholars, despite their disproportionate presence.[6] In 1883 the publication of the first *Australasian Medical Directory* was welcomed by a *Glasgow Medical Journal* reviewer who praised the 'great enterprise and practical sense' of the promoters; it also, he stated confidently, offered proof that the Australasians were well on their way to being a united profession.[7]

Doubts must remain as to how accurate or comprehensive the *Directory* really was, given the federal structure of Australia at this time and the problem of maintaining lines of communication. The *Directory* is invaluable, however, in providing the first measure by which to quantify and analyse the medical profession in Australasia since colonisation began almost a century before.

Of the 1545 practitioners registered in 1883, 649 (42 per cent) possessed Scottish qualifications, compared with 739 (47.8 per cent) who had English degrees or diplomas. Holders of Irish qualifications totalled 261 (16.9 per cent). Relative to population ratio — approximately 1:10 in the case of Scotland: England — these are very obviously disproportionate totals. Before leaping to conclusions, observers should take heed of the fact that possession of Scottish qualifications gives no indication of nationality. Of 8,262 British medical degrees recorded in the first half of the 19th century, almost 8,000 — a staggering 96 per cent — were awarded by one or other of the four Scottish Universities.[8] This figure inevitably declined as London and English provincial universities strengthened and expanded their medical schools.

Despite these changes, it has recently been calculated that in 1883 only 37 per cent of registered medical practitioners in New South Wales were university graduates, of whom just under half had qualified in Scotland.[9] Such computations reveal only part of the true picture. Many of those who went to practice in Australasia were equipped with the licentiate or fellowship diplomas of the Colleges north and south of the border, or in Ireland. Some, to confuse the issue further, were possessed of both degrees and diplomas, often from entirely separate schools. Almost one-third of the Scottish registrands (204 from 649) also boasted English qualifications; a further 54 had both Scottish and Irish certificates; eight had gone so far as to register degrees or diplomas from all three countries.

One useful indication of the respective influence of the four Scottish centres may be obtained from a further subdivision of the 649 Scottish-trained men who registered in 1882. Of these, more than two-thirds (452 from 649) held Edinburgh qualifications. Glasgow accounted for exactly one-quarter (162) while Aberdeen (59) and St Andrews (39)[10] brought up the rear. This concentration is readily explained by the existence of extra-mural schools in Edinburgh and Glasgow, together with the Royal Colleges of Physicians and Surgeons in the former and the Faculty of Physicians and Surgeons in the latter.

Enticing as they are, it is dangerous to read too much into these figures. The successful interpretation of such data, however sophisticated, depends also upon a qualitative assessment. In the first *Australasian Medical Dictionary* of 1883, Dr Robert Scot Skirving, an Edinburgh graduate of 1881, was recorded as 'travelling in Queensland'. Impressed with what he found, Scot Skirving settled in Australia. Forty years later he presented his recollections of that period at a meeting of the New South Wales Branch of the British Medical Association (BMA). In 1883, he claimed, Sydney had a population of 273,400 served by 186 doctors, not one of whom had received his education in the city. By 1925, on the other hand, more than two-thirds of the city's practitioners had been educated locally. It was not only in the sphere of medical education that things had changed, according to the venerable doctor:

> 'In the early 'eighties it was not difficult to earn a living as a doctor. Any sober, honest doctor of fair abilities could always get a practice in New South Wales. I could not say the same today'.[11]

Scot Skirving's bullish view of the past must be treated with caution. Even in the decade of which he spoke, the Antipodean medical scene was apparently becoming more competitive. In March 1884 the New Zealand correspondent of the *Glasgow Medical Journal* warned that:

> 'No bright youth from the old country needs come here with the hope of enlightening us, or thinking to secure an excellent city practice. The man who will be successful here is the strong able-bodied general practitioner, fit for a country practice'[12]

The time described in their various ways by these two men was a period of expansion in the Australasian colonies, reflected in an increased demand for doctors. Of 170 Glasgow medical graduates who worked in Australia prior to 1897, no fewer than 71 had qualified after 1880, with 55 of these graduating during that decade.[13] Any attempt to explain this pattern is dependent on factors other than the simply numerical: it is probable that career destination was influenced by calibre of degree and the extent of competition both at home and abroad; the time lapse between qualification and arrival in Australasia may alter the historian's assessment of the bald statistics quoted above; the accurate recording of place of origin and country of birth of these 'Scottish' practitioners would undoubtedly reveal many Englishmen and Irishmen, and not a few Australians or New Zealanders, in the ranks of the 'Scottish' graduates, diplomates and fellows.

Any failure to give due weight to such factors is understandable at a distance of some 11,000 miles. Few historians can claim a degree of familiarity with archival sources in both continents and it is all too easy to be lured into error. A recent Oxford DPhil thesis described Dr James Jamieson as an 'Anglo-Australian gynaecologist',[14] despite the fact that Jamieson was a native of Beith in Ayrshire and received his medical education in Glasgow before emigrating to Australia. Jamieson's nationality was restored in 1985 in a footnote to an admirable short biography by Diana Dyason, a leading Australian historian of medicine.[15] Even Dyason's study, dependent as it was on Jamieson's own writings and local Australian sources, erred occasionally. The honours MD was first awarded at Glasgow in 1845, but Jamieson's name does not appear on the list of recipients, as claimed in Dyason's 'crude chronology' of the man.[16] According to the same source, Jamieson's father was a furniture manufacturer, but the entries in the University matriculation albums, written in the future doctor's own hand, describe him as a seed merchant. Perhaps most misleading of all for a current reader, Jamieson was described as MD MS, both now recognised as postgraduate awards. James Jamieson actually graduated MD CM, and at a time when these were still first or undergraduate degrees.

The case of James Jamieson demonstrates another problem for cross-cultural historians, that of racial stereotyping. Describing Jamieson's talents in his history of the Melbourne Medical School, KF Russell noted that he taught clinical medicine with 'Scottish thoroughness at the bedside'.[17] Similar characteristics were identified by another

Australasian medical historian, Dr Wright St-Clair, who attributed the development of the University of Otago medical school in the 1870s to the endeavours of John Halliday Scott, foundation professor of Anatomy and an Edinburgh graduate who 'With Scottish thoroughness . . . set quietly about establishing a school on the model that he knew from Edinburgh'.[18]

Scott was also the target for a rather different, and less flattering, expression of a perceived national trait. DWC Jones, the first chronicler of the Otago School, described Scott's success as based in large measure on his 'Scottish care of the bawbees'.[19] It is not difficult to cite other examples of this type, such as Professor Russell's claim that John Henry MacFarland, Chancellor of Melbourne University in the early part of this century, managed its affairs with 'Scottish frugality'.[20] Tom Brooking, a New Zealand historian with a particular interest in dentistry, cites dour 'puritanism and canniness' as the popularly-held distinguishing features of the 19th century immigrants from Scotland,[21] suggesting that such views are general rather than particular. This vision is perhaps best expressed by Eric Richards. Assessing the existing literature on the Scots in Australia, primarily with non-Australian readers in mind, Richards summarised the conventional Australian perception, of such immigrants as that of the 'canny, pertinaceous, calculating, dour, upwardly mobile Scot'.[22]

Coupled with the continued acceptance of these cultural stereotypes described by Richards and others, there appears to be a puzzling lack of curiosity concerning the background and training of those doctors who comprised the great majority of the Australasian medical profession in the 19th century. At the 1933 inaugural meeting of the Historical Section of the Victoria Branch of the BMA, Dr GT Howard delivered a paper on Port Phillip's Early Doctors, in celebration of the settlement of the colony in 1835. In the course of his address the speaker made the following observation:

> 'John Sproat, LRCS (Edinburgh) 1824, MD (Edinburgh) 1828, arrived in Melbourne in 1838 or 1839 and left finally for Scotland in 1854. He was evidently an unobtrusive person as there is practically no other record of his present'.[23]

In fact, it was not at all difficult, using the UK *Medical Directories*, to discover that Sproat died at home in Scotland in August 1856.[24] Unobtrusive they may have been in terms of publications or as leaders of the profession, but these 19th century Australasian doctors are by no means inaccessible.

Given the wealth of information contained in matriculation albums, student class lists, examination registers and other Scottish University records, it is both surprising and disappointing that so few prosopographical studies have been attempted in the half century since the formation of this early medical history society.[25] With the advent of easier access to the creation and exploitation of machine-readable databases, the prospects of closer collaboration between Australian and UK scholars in this field have increased significantly. Hopefully, some of the pitfalls outlined in this section of the paper may thus be avoided.

While the collective picture is important, there is still a great deal to be learned from the study of individual doctors. In estimating the extent of the 'Scottish' impact it may be helpful to invoke the 'nature-nurture' model, which emerges from the debate as to whether cultural and environmental background play a greater role than genetic influence in determining subsequent development. Nowhere is this better illustrated in a medical history context than in the transfer of antiseptic surgery to Australia.

Joseph Lister's dramatic inception of antisepsis at the Glasgow Royal Infirmary in the 1860s is too well-known to require further elaboration at this juncture. Paradoxically, in view of what follows, Lister was not himself a Scot, but almost all of his early supporters in Australia were Scots-born, or had received their medical education north of the border. Lister arrived in Edinburgh in the autumn of 1853 as house surgeon in Professor James Syme's wards in the Royal Infirmary. In the course of the next few months the young surgeon established lasting friendships with six of the dressers in the Infirmary, including George Hogarth Pringle.[26] After service in the Crimea and with the Cunard and P & O steamship lines, latterly working between Suez and Sydney, Pringle established himself in practice at Parramatta in New South Wales in 1860.[27]

The publication in *The Lancet* in March 1867 of Lister's account of his new antiseptic procedures brought a sharp divide between those who hailed it as a long-awaited breakthrough and the sceptics or traditionalists. Australia was then some 3-4 months by sea from the UK. Although telegraphic communication between London and Calcutta had been reduced to some five hours in 1863, the cable link to Australia, which brought that continent into direct contact with 'the grand electric chain which united all the nations of the earth', was not completed until October 1872.[28] In any event, it is doubtful if details of the complex and revolutionary methods could have been conveyed satisfactorily by cable. Despite these drawbacks, Pringle had adopted antiseptic techniques by October 1867, and never wavered in his support for his former colleague thereafter, going so far as to publicise his endeavours in the lay press, in the absence of local medical journals or societies.[29]

In Melbourne, the introduction of antisepsis was carried out by William Gillbee. Although registered as a Member of the Royal College of Surgeons of England, Gillbee had spent the years 1844 to 1847 as a medical student in Edinburgh, before completing his training at Guy's Hospital in London. He later returned to Edinburgh in 1851 for postgraduate study. Gillbee thus witnessed at first hand the excitement and sense of local achievement when JY Simpson pioneered the use of chloroform anesthesia in January 1847. It is difficult to quantify the extent of Gillbee's future loyalty to his *alma mater*, but it is arguable that this made him particularly receptive to further innovations from the Edinburgh School.[30]

In 1966-7 David O'Sullivan penned two articles in the *Medical Journal of Australia* to co-incide with the centenary of the antiseptic revolution.[31] In one of these articles O'Sullivan argued that Gillbee's ready acceptance of Listerian doctrine occurred because 'His distance from the Glasgow scene allowed him to be untrammelled by local prejudice, and his Scottish training would remove any scepticism'.[32] My own interpretation would be that a Scottish education, particularly for those who came under Lister's influence, rather encouraged a questioning and sceptical approach. As for local prejudice, it is true that many of Lister's most vigorous critics were his fellow Glasgow surgeons; it is equally true, however, that Lister's 1860s students were among his most loyal supporters, and it was this group which carried the new gospel world-wide.

In Canada, the word was spread by Archibald Malloch, formerly a house surgeon in Glasgow Royal;[33] in Australia, the carbolic spray was introduced in 1872 by Edwin Hinchcliffe who graduated from Edinburgh in 1870[34] — the first year of Lister's tenure of the Chair of Surgery there; in New Zealand, Listerism was promoted by Dr John Rutherford Ryley[35], who obtained the Licentiateship of the Royal College of Surgeons of Edinburgh in 1862 and the Fellowship five years later. Incidental to this major theme, Ryley illustrates another of the recurring problems in determining the impact of Scotland on Australasian medicine. According to O'Sullivan, Ryley claimed to have studied under Lister during the latter's first two sessions in Glasgow. There is, however, no evidence that Ryley attended any University classes in Glasgow, nor does his name appear in the list of Lister's GRI students. Clearly, the validation of such an assertion was no more certain in 1966 than it had been a century earlier.

George Pringle, arguably the original disciple, died at sea in 1872 while homeward bound for Scotland.[36] His son, James Hogarth Pringle, returned to Scotland from Australia and qualified in medicine at Edinburgh in 1885. Within a few years he had become assistant to William Macewen at the Glasgow Royal Infirmary, where the two men made a formidable surgical team.[37] Macewen, an early supporter of Lister, was largely responsible for the evolution from antiseptic to aseptic surgery; as such, he was an obvious focal point for the young Scots-Australian surgeon come home to follow in his father's footsteps. In addition, Macewen already had Australian links of his own. His eldest brother, Thomas, had settled in Queensland during the 1850s goldrush while his sister Janet was married and living in Sydney.[38]

As immediate Past President of the BMA Sir William, as he had become, attended the 1st Australasian Medical Conference in 1923. One of his first acts on arriving at Sydney was to pay a call on George Hogarth Pringle's widow, now a very frail old lady. Macewen's letters home also record several convivial evenings spent in the company of former Glasgow students.[39]

One of those who entertained Sir William was Dr Charles Duguid of Adelaide. A fervent supporter of Aboriginal rights, Duguid zealously promoted the surgical techniques which he had learned from Macewen as student and house surgeon. In 1957, three years after attending the BMA annual meeting in Glasgow, Duguid, now the last surviving house surgeon from the Macewen era, published an affectionate and glowing tribute to his former Chief.[40] The Apostolic Succession, through Lister, Pringle, Macewen, Pringle and Duguid thus stretched over two continents and more than a century.

If the preceding paragraphs suggest a particular Scottish dimension attached to the progress of surgery in Australia, the same may be said of radiology, where Scotland, and especially Glasgow, had a considerable influence on developments in Australia after Rontgen's discovery of the new X-rays in 1895. Such involvement is not surprising when we recollect that Lord Kelvin was then Professor of Natural Philosophy at Glasgow University and was one of the first to be informed of Rontgen's work. Incapacitated with a leg injury at the time, Kelvin encouraged his assistant and nephew, JT Bottomley, to investigate the rays in conjunction with Lord Blythswoood — a gifted amateur physicist — and Dr John Macintyre, medical electrician to the Royal Infirmary. As a result of this activity, the GRI established the world's first hospital radiology department in February 1896.[41]

News of this innovative technology reached the Australian public through the pages of the *Sydney Daily Telegraph* on 31 January 1896 and the first Australian X-ray photograph was taken on 3 March. These and the other details of early advances appear in *Salute to the X-Ray Pioneers of Australia*, published in 1946.[42] Surprisingly, the author of Salute makes no reference to the disproportionate contribution of Scottish-trained men amongst the medically-qualified pioneers. A cursory glance at the *Medical Directory* would have revealed that more than half of these men possessed Scottish degrees, almost all of which had been obtained during the 1880s. Such a course of action would also have explained the initial interest of Charles Johnston, who 'happened to be visiting Britain at the time of Rontgen's announcement'.[43] In fact, Johnston was in the final year of his medical studies at Edinburgh University, from whence he graduated MB CM in 1896.

Salute also recorded that Dr BM Quaife donated £100 to Sydney Hospital 'for the purpose of obtaining the most perfect apparatus for the practical production of X-rays to be used in the diagnosis of disease and injury in the interests of suffering humanity'.[44] In reality, the donor was Dr Frederick Harrison Quaife, son of a Presbyterian Minister and a New Zealander by birth, who studied under Lister in Glasgow and graduated in 1867. He maintained contact with a number of his Glasgow contemporaries over the years and may have been encouraged in his radiological venture as a result. It is perhaps relevant that his younger brother, William, also a Glasgow medical graduate, was a near contemporary of John Macintyre and of Dr Donald Mackintosh, another Glasgow pioneer who published an *Atlas of Skiagraphy* in 1899.[45]

The Centenary Book of the University of Sydney Faculty of Medicine suggests yet another stimulus to Quaife's involvement, stating that Quaife went initially to Glasgow to study physics under Kelvin, before eventually switching to medicine.[46] According to the compilers of this large but somewhat erratic volume, Quaife's interest in physics remains an enigma; it became even more so with my failure to find any evidence that Quaife attended Kelvin's classes. His four years of study, from 1863 to 1867, are fully documented in the University registers and class lists, but nowhere does physics appear in his curriculum. Once again it seems we should revise the authorised version.[47]

Kelvin's influence is easier to substantiate in the case of one of the other leading Australian figures, WJ Hancock. Hancock was the nephew of James Thomson, brother of Lord Kelvin and Professor of Civil Engineering in the University of Glasgow. For two years — not four as he later claimed in his 1906 application for membership of the Institution of Civil Engineers — Hancock studied under his uncle. He subsequently emigrated to Australia where he became Superintendent of Telephones in Western Australia. Recognising the importance of Rontgen's discovery in 1896, Hancock acquired suitable equipment from the London Hospital and began to provide a radiological service to Perth Public Hospital, a post which he retained in a purely honorary capacity for more than two decades.[48]

Ironically, in view of my criticism of Dr Moscucci's 'Anglo-Australian gynaecologist', Kelvin, his brother James, JT Bottomley and WJ Hancock were all born in Ireland, although educated primarily in Scotland. Regardless of this co-incidence of nationality, it is arguable that their influence on Australia was essentially 'Scottish'.

The complexities suggested in this paper confirm the need for a reappraisal of Scotland's contribution to Antipodean medicine. In October 1953 'The Section of Medical History of the Victorian Branch of the British Medical Association' was formed as the successor to the long-defunct body addressed by Dr Howard in 1933.[49] The catalyst which sparked this revival was the imminent arrival in Australia of Dr Douglas Guthrie, founder in 1948 of the Scottish Society of the History of Medicine. Guthrie's visit stimulated a widespread interest in the subject. Four years later Dr Bryan Gandevia of Sydney published an article on 'The Pattern of Australian Medical History', prefaced by an apt quotation from one of Guthrie's works:

> '. . . the writer [of a history of medicine] may be tempted to exaggerate the importance of great discoveries and to lay great stress on the lives of famous men. It should be remembered that this is only one aspect of history, a survey of peaks and not of the valleys, a study of the milestones rather than of the miles between'[50]

Guthrie's words can be taken, on one level, as a plea for the kind of prosopographical study referred to earlier in this paper. It is therefore appropriate to conclude with a second quotation from this source. On 15 March 1985 the *Medical Journal of Australia* announced the foundation of a Medical History Society of Australia under the heading 'History of Medicine — a phoenix rising'. Commenting on this welcome development the Editor Emeritus, Ronald Winton, chose once more to express his thoughts in the words of Dr Guthrie. 'Seemingly', he wrote, 'they see the force of Douglas Guthrie's dictum: "History, despite all its failures and inconsistencies, remains the foundation of today's knowledge and the basis of tomorrow's discoveries."'

Despite — or perhaps more forcibly because of — its failures and inconsistencies, I hope this paper may encourage both Scottish and Antipodean medical historians to respond to the obvious need for increased dialogue in order to promote a more accurate assessment of the dual relationship of Scottish and Australian medicine.

Postscript

On delivering this paper I was gently chastised by Professor Harold Attwood of Melbourne, a participant at the 11th British Congress on the History of Medicine, for prematurity. One of his responsibilities while in Britain, he informed me, was to obtain legal guidance on the constitution of the nascent society. It gives me great pleasure to record that his mission was successful, and that The Australian Society of the History of Medicine was formally established, under the Presidency of Dr Bryan Gandevia, at the Third National Conference on Medical History and Health in Australia, held in Adelaide from 23-25 November 1986.

American Jewish Medical Students in Scotland 1925-40

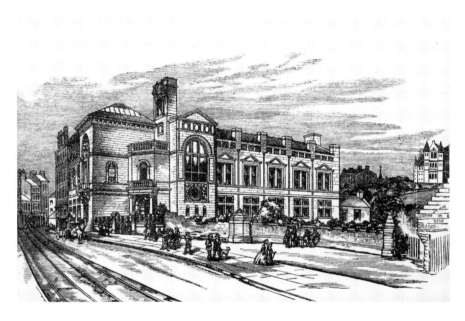

Anderson's College Medical School at the time of its opening in 1888. The College survived as an independent body until 1947, when it was absorbed by the University of Glasgow.

Chapter 11

American Jewish Medical Students in Scotland 1925-40

K E Collins

One fascinating story in the history of medical education in Scotland concerns the hundreds of Americans who made their way to the Scottish medical schools between 1925 and 1940. The majority came in the late 1930s when Scotland was the most popular overseas destination for Americans studying medicine abroad. At a time when thousands of American medical students are again finding their way to foreign medical schools, it is of value to examine the reasons for this pre-war phenomenon.

Medical graduations in Scotland, which had peaked in the early 1920s, fell steadily during the rest of the decade. The high figures after the First World War can be explained on the basis of war-time disruption and the subsequent fall in student numbers points to the quantity of surplus capacity in the Scottish medical schools. These trends are particularly clear in the large medical schools at the universities in Glasgow and Edinburgh while, as will be seen, there were additional factors at play in the smaller medical schools in Aberdeen and St Andrews.

From the start of the 1930s other factors became increasingly important, some with major international implications. Firstly, the demand from local students for places in medicine was rising steadily and there were increasing signs of international interest in Scottish medical study, initially from the United States and later from Central Europe. While these two geographical locations were to provide the major centres from which medical students came to Scotland during the 1930s, there were smaller but still significant numbers from countries like Egypt, Nigeria, India and Ceylon. In the 1930s the output from the various Scottish medical schools made up over one-third of the entire UK total. The number of overseas students dominated the output of St Andrews University and the extra-mural medical schools in Glasgow and Edinburgh and represented a significant element amongst the graduates of Edinburgh University.

The difficulty of Jews in gaining admission to some of the leading medical schools in the United States was being commented on by 1929. In November of that year Professor Frank Gavin of the General Theological Seminary said that the level of discrimination had become so intense that many American Jews were being forced to study overseas, especially in Scotland.[1] This difficulty was also remarked upon at the same time at the conference of the Association of American Medical Colleges by the Dean of the St Louis University School of Medicine, Dr AM Schwitella.[2]

There were differences in attitude to this perceived anti-Jewish discrimination in America and various solutions were suggested. Better vocational counselling to suggest alternative career possibilities and the establishment of a Jewish medical school were recommended. Various Jewish voices were also raised, claiming that increasing the numbers of Jewish physicians would produce anti-semitism and could be damaging to the interests of the Jews in America.[3] As long as the Jews constituted only a small percentage of the population they could not represent any threat to established practitioners. By the 1920s the children of the large Eastern European immigration to America at the turn of the century were beginning to move into the professions. Between 1880 and 1925 there had been a rapid expansion of higher education in the United States and there were places for all who had the appropriate entrance qualifications. Before 1920 the only criterion for college entry had been educational success, but in the following years character tests and psychological assessments were introduced and these were 'arbitrarily made to serve the end desired'.[4]

The First World War unleashed passions of racial and religious prejudice in America and immigration quotas were introduced which restricted places for those from Southern and Eastern Europe, thus reserving more places for those of British and Scandinavian stock. The universitites appeared to be seeking to introduce the same criteria for selection of students as the nation was doing with respect to the character of its future citizens.[5] While most universities were reticent about their possession of a restrictive entry quota, Harvard was quite open about its limitation of Jewish students during the presidency of Lawrence Lowell.[6] Lowell felt that Jewish students posed a threat to the homogeneity of the Harvard student body and a 'Sifting Committee' was established which openly limited Jewish students. Allowing Jews to compete for places on a basis of equality with other candidates was thought to be likely to provoke intense race feeling.

At Columbia, Jewish enrolment fell due to the application of intelligence and psychological tests from 40% in 1919 to only half of that two years later.[7] At Princeton one of the factors reducing the numbers of Jewish students was the prospect of social isolation on a campus where eating clubs dominated undergraduate life.[8] Rutgers University attempted to introduce a Jewish quota by limiting Jewish entry to a percentage similar to the ethnic composition of the State of New Jersey.[9] When a complaint was made in 1930 to the New Jersey State Board of Regents, an assurance was given that Rutgers had no intention to apply discriminatory processes.

The restrictions placed on Jewish students entering college also applied at medical schools. The catalyst for change in American medicine was the Flexner Report of 1910,[10] which pointed to the large number of second-rate medical institutions, and the inevitable reduction in medical places was designed to lead to an improvement in standards. However, it also became the excuse for the exclusion of Jews, women, negroes and Italians from medical school.[11] In December 1930, Dr Harold Rypins, himself a Jew and the Secretary of the New York State Board of Medical Examiners, pointed out that there were only 6,000 freshman places and double that number of applicants.[12] He insisted that the difficulty faced by Jewish students was based on lack of space and geographical factors. He did acknowledge that although Jews made up 17% of medical students nationally, a large number of suitably qualified applicants were being excluded. The Jewish students themselves were under no illusions about the existence of such a quota, and the failure of exceptionally well qualified candidates to gain medical school places reinforced this. Julius Axelrod, 1970 Nobel Prizewinner for Biochemistry, was denied access to medical school in 1933 and George Rosen, doyen of medical historians, failed to enter medical school despite a good college career and obtained a place to study medicine in Germany.[13]

The difficulties were most intense for Jewish New Yorkers and almost all the Americans studying in Scotland came from there. While the Jewish students were not alone in facing discrimination they showed the greatest ingenuity in finding alternative careers.[14] Some turned to dentistry. While only a few of the excluded Italians found their way to Italian medical schools, for the dejected and rejected Jew the way abroad was the best prospect. During the 1930s increasing numbers of Americans studied abroad, especially in Scotland, Italy, Austria, Germany and Switzerland. By 1934 the Scottish contingent was the largest of the overseas groups of American students and the Scottish proportion increased as anti-semitism became more marked in Germany, Austria and Italy.[15]

Citizens of the USA Enrolled in Faculties of Medicine Abroad

	1930-31	31-32	32-33	33-34	34-35	35-36	36-37	37-38	38-39
Austria	114	175	271	253	235	183	185	172	—
England	52	61	57	69	78	60	47	29	36
France	25	62	78	86	89	75	40	11	18
Germany	72	189	439	331	246	204	245	87	45
Ireland	14	21	20	4	6	7	7	4	9
Italy	78	155	282	258	286	265	265	214	54
Scotland	256	286	416	444	476	369	386	525	401
Switzerland	65	214	405	351	396	366	316	123	56
others	34	43	84	107	125	108	140	133	61
TOTAL	710	1206	2052	1903	1937	1637	1631	1298	680

Source: Jou. Amer, Med. Soc. (1939), Vol *113,* 772

Jewish students were irritated by the attempts of the American medical authorities to denigrate their standards and to deny them the opportunity of studying abroad, while removing their chances of studying at home. The Jewish quota was not presented in an anti-semitic way so that it could be claimed that the aim was to improve standards by reducing the numbers of students. The reality was that Jewish students faced restrictions with the adoption of admissions' procedures which discriminated against them in subtle ways.

During the 1930s the American Medical Association called for a further reduction in the number of medical school places.[16] This resulted in a further reduction in the number of Jews studying medicine. Again Jewish New Yorkers were especially affected, caught as they were between geographic quotas which sought to limit ethnic entry to medical schools and out-of-town quotas which applied at national institutions. Medicine was seen by Jews as the first career choice because of the status and security it offered and because of the high regard for medicine in the Jewish tradition. Jewish families were prepared to make considerable financial sacrifices to put their sons through medical school. Given this Jewish obsession with medicine it was unrealistic to expect that Jewish medical school enrolments could be held to the level of their proportion in the general population.

At Cornell University the proportion of Jewish students at the medical school fell from 25% in 1930 to 10% ten years later.[17] At Columbia University medical school the drop was even greater — from 33% in 1930 to 10% only a few years later.[18] These restrictions made it particularly difficult for the graduates of City College New York, which had a predominantly Jewish roll, to find medical school places. At the Yale University medical school, the Dean (Milton Charles Winternitz) created an admissions' committee in 1930 which had the detailed instructions: 'never admit more than 5 Jews, take only two Italian Catholics and take no blacks at all'.[19] Winternitz admitted that over 50% of the applicants to the medical school were Jewish but that the percentage admitted never rose above 10%. He felt that it would be 'unwise to permit the student body to include an unduly large proportion of any racial and religious group'. The school of medicine had to maintain the representative balance of the population it served. Winternitz's successor continued this policy and the 1938-9 report showed that, while 28% of qualified non-Jewish doctors applicants received a place, only 3% of similarly qualified Jews gained entry. At least one admissions' committee record from this period shows that applicants were grouped under three headings: 'Women', 'Americans' and 'Hebrews'.

There were fears in America during the 1930s that the medical profession was becoming overcrowded. Dean Willard Rappleye of Columbia University said at the Minneapolis meeting of the Association of American Colleges in 1933 that there was no need for a large number of physicians because of increased urbanisation, improved transportation and preventive medicine.[20] Voices suggesting that America was unlikely to become overdoctored were in a distinct minority.

Jewish students faced other disadvantages which gave them a lower priority in finding medical school places. With an immigrant background few could claim 'medical heritage', that is having a parent who had studied medicine. Few Jewish parents had the resources to make available endowment funds which might have enticed the medical schools to find a place for their son. Indeed, many did not have the funds to turn to private out-of-date medical schools if turned down for a place in their own State. It might even be cheaper to study in Scotland. The round trip from the States cost $100 and digs could be obtained for about $7.50 per week. Monthly expenses were generally about $75.[21] Inclusive of fees, which varied from £120 for the course at St Mungo's College in Glasgow to £250 for the course at the Universities of Glasgow and Aberdeen, the annual costs came to about $1300 (£260).[22] While this budget did not allow for luxuries, it was adequate. The American students were deeply offended by the novelist Jerome Weidman's portrayal of a New York medical student in Edinburgh who had a very negative attitude to his studies and who lived in 'a dirty old tenement with an evil-smelling hallway'.[23] Most students were too conscious of the financial sacrifices being made at home on their behalf to neglect their studies.

Because the Americans had all attended college prior to their studying in Scotland, they were a few years older than the local students and that much more mature. They were well motivated to learn and complete their studies and they proved to be a formidable challenge at examination times for the Scottish students. They were certainly not 'second-rate' as the American medical authorities claimed.[24] The Americans at St Andrews won their due share of class prizes and certificates. At the University of Glasgow the 1934 Brunton Prize, for the most distinguished graduate, was won by an American as was the West of Scotland Prize. Indeed, no less than six out of the eleven Americans graduating at the University of Glasgow in 1934 did so with honours or with commendation. The lecturers at the Royal Colleges medical school in Edinburgh also recognised the educational attainments of their American students and confirmed this in a letter to Dr Zapffe, the Secretary of the Association of American Medical Colleges, in 1931.

The restrictive entry practices remained in force until after the Second World War when they began to yield slowly to the pressure of public criticism. There was opposition to the quota from Jewish war veterans and, aided by the increase in the numbers of medical school places and a drop in the level of applications, there was a three to four-fold increase in Jewish enrolment in medical colleges by 1956.[25]

American interest in medical study in Britain can be identified from about 1926. This trend came to the attention of the General Medical Council during 1930 when it was stated that over 250 prospective students had been turned away from the Universities of Birmingham and Manchester.[26] A memorandum was prepared by the Registrar of the Council on the question of American medical students. The Americans had registered their concern about the matter because they felt that if students who had been deemed unsuitable in the States could obtain qualifications abroad then difficulties over medical standards would ensue. It was acknowledged that those seeking places in Britain had varying levels of qualifications and it was agreed that it was important to ensure that any Americans admitted to British medical schools should have attained an adequate standard in their pre-clinical studies in college. After some correspondence between the GMC and the National Board of Medical Examiners in the States, it was agreed that students intending to enter medical school in Britain should produce evidence of their eligibility by producing a satisfactory collegiate record. It had been acknowledged by Dr WC Rappleye, Director of Studies of the Commission on Medical Examination organised by the American Medical Colleges and who had been present at meetings of the GMC in May 1930, that in fact the most common reason for students not being accepted into American medical schools was that the schools were designated as 'class full'. This was said to be the least objectionable designation by which students could be rejected on personal or racial grounds.

The GMC realised that it was treading on dangerous ground as the Medical Act did not cover admission to medical school in the pre-clinical stage and the Council did not wish to interfere with the prerogatives of the British medical schools. Concern was also expressed that in view of the reciprocal arrangements in existence that British medical schools should not permit Americans to obtain their qualifications in a shorter time than would have been possible in the States.

The Scottish Branch of the GMC also had several meetings during 1930 to discuss admission procedures for the American applicants. At one of these meetings Dr JS Rodman, Secretary of the National Board of Medical Examiners of the USA, was present by invitation. It was recommended that all applications from America for admission to medical schools in Scotland should be forwarded to the Registrar of the Scottish Branch Council for verification of authenticity. It was noted at the November meeting of the Scottish Branch in 1930 that some twenty Americans had applied under the new arrangements and had been accepted for study. These arrangements proved satisfactory and in the 1932 Presidential Address to the General Medical Council it was stated that the previous difficulties had almost completely disappeared and that the Council was particularly indebted to Dr Zapffe, of the Association of American Medical Colleges, for his 'untiring help in regard to verification and evaluation of certificates'.[27] The President was also pleased to note the cordial references in the Association's own journal in the States to the part played by the GMC in dealing with these matters.

The great majority of Americans studying in Britain came to Scotland, with the Scottish preponderance increasing through the 1930s. The initial trend was for the Americans to enter the universities in the late 1920s and early 1930s but by 1935 the move was towards the extra-mural medical schools which lay outwith the authority of the universities.

At the University of Glasgow there were 23 American applicants for the 1928-9 session. In January 1929 it was decided to fix the capacity of the medical school at 200 per annum and as numbers fell below this level over the next three or four sessions it was possible to admit a number of Americans — between seven and fifteen — each year. The Medical Faculty of the University of Glasgow took note of the decisions of the GMC in 1930 but decided to continue to make selections of American students as before.

By 1932, the number of American applications was rising steadily and there was a clear need for a more critical selection policy. The Clerk to the Faculty, who was processing an increasing number of applications, was instructed in November 1932 that, with a limited number of places and increasing demand from home students, there was no likelihood of overseas students being accepted. Senate records show that 66 Americans applied in 1932 and that 250 foreign applications were received in 1935, without specifying country of origin.

The admissions' policy in Edinburgh University differed only slightly but took into account Edinburgh's tradition of being an international university. The topic of American admissions was first discussed in 1928 when the Medical Faculty set up a committee to discuss the question. This committee functioned as a clearing house for the processing of applications and did not adjudicate on the question of whether foreign students should be admitted. The committee finally made a report in 1934 and there was agreement on limiting annual admissions to 220. Preference for overseas admissions was to be given to students from the Colonies, especially from areas like the British West Indies which did not have medical schools of their own. There was to be a limit of 10% on students from Commonwealth countries like Australia, New Zealand, South Africa and India. Students would be admitted from China if 'well qualified' and from Egypt and the United States if 'exceptionally well qualified'. Thus a few Americans continued to be admitted.

In St Andrews University a considerable number of Americans studied medicine from 1927. The peak year for American graduates was 1933 when 31 of the 46 graduands were American, and all but two of them were from New York or New Jersey. In the ten years preceding the first graduation of Americans, St Andrews medical classes had been very small with on average less than 30 doctors graduating each year. However, even after the number of Americans in St Andrews declined, the University was able to maintain its increased number of medical students.

This remarkably large group of American students, who studied in St Andrews and took their clinical course in Dundee, formed almost one-third of all the students between 1932 and 1937. It is thought that Sir Charles Irvine, who was a frequent visitor to the States, encouraged the Americans to come when he learned of the difficulties faced by prospective Jewish medical students.[28] New Yorkers were also attracted by a Scottish science lecturer at New York University.[29] Frank Charteris, then Dean of the Medical Faculty, was also supportive of the Americans and he nurtured their attachment to the University.[30] The American graduates showed their appreciation by forming the St Andrews American Medical Alumni Association which has raised thousands of dollars for St Andrews University to endow scholarships and provide other academic support.

The primary consideration in Aberdeen was the provision of places for local students, although a group of eleven Americans was admitted in 1928. The rising level of local applicants meant that not all qualified applicants from the Aberdeen area could be admitted. In 1930 alone Aberdeen University received no less than 203 medical applications from America, with virtually all the candidates being graduates of the College of the City of New York and New York University.

Of the three Scottish extra-mural schools the smallest was St Mungo's College, located at the Glasgow Royal Infirmary. The Medical Faculty there was concerned at the low level of enrolments, totalling less than 100 students in 1927-8. They considered amalgamation with Anderson's College, the other Glasgow extra-mural school, but Anderson's College did not favour such a move. With the arrival of the Americans the student roll began to increase dramatically. In 1936-7 St Mungo's agreed to admit about 100 Americans for the winter and summer sessions and to charge them a deposit of £5.

Anderson's College, which was situated near Glasgow's Western Infirmary, was a larger institution than St Mungo's. Some university students were attracted to those classes where the teaching was of an exceptionally high standard, such as in anatomy and physiology. Despite the huge influx of Americans to Anderson's College, the numbers reaching over 250 in 1938, there are no references in the College minutes concerning the admission of the Americans. The University of Glasgow was alarmed at the strain the number of foreign students was placing on teaching facilities in the city and it suggested in 1937 that the extra-mural colleges adopt the same admissions' policy as the University.

Anderson's College and St Mungo's both decided not to admit any Americans for the session commencing in October 1939 but the outbreak of war meant that no new students were able to arrive anyway. There was continuing resentment amongst the honorary clinical staff at the University about the success of the extra-mural colleges in recruiting so many foreign students with the accompanying prosperity this implied. Extra-mural college lecturers received class fees from their students and handed a proportion over to the college authorities.

The medical school of the two Royal Colleges in Edinburgh also based its considerable student enrolment on recruitment of foreign students. In 1932, the 36 Americans were only four fewer than the British students, while there were also some Egyptian, Chinese, South African and Indian students. In 1930 the medical school developed a system for the processing of American applications to ensure that the Americans had the correct entry qualifications. While they would supply information on American student admissions to the American medical authorities, they reserved for themselves the full responsibility for admissions. The medical school continued to admit substantial numbers of Americans through the 1930s and did not suffer any limitation in numbers following discussions with the University of Edinburgh about the maximum medical teaching capacity in the city. As in Glasgow, the outbreak of war brought the influx of Americans to an end as all who had planned to start their courses in October 1939 were unable to come.

Some American medical students who had not completed their courses by 1939 were dismayed by the news that the New York and New Jersey State Boards of Examiners planned not to recognise the Scottish Triple Qualification, which was the final examination of the extra-mural colleges. However, it was subsequently made clear that the ruling was not retrospective and would not apply to students who had already started their courses in Scotland.[31]

Students who were in America for the summer vacation in 1939 were faced with the prospect of being refused permission to return to Scotland to complete their studies as the US State Department had discontinued the issuing of visas to combat areas.[32] Following popular pressure from the specially formed American Medical Clubs of Scotland, supported by the Mayor of New York and other personalities, it was agreed late in 1939 that students in the last two years of their studies should be allowed to return to Scotland. Fifty students returned to Scotland but there were more than 300 who were at earlier stages of their course. The numbers of Americans taking the Triple Qualification fell from 80 in 1940 to 27 in 1942 and then averaged about ten over the next five years. The Americans studying in Scotland had a good record in passing State Board examinations on returning home. The best results were obtained by Glasgow University's American graduates who achieved 100% success in New York State Board examinations. A number of others did manage to return to Scotland after the war to complete their studies and a few managed to find places in America or in neutral Switzerland. By the 1950s there was only a handful of American medical students in Scotland. For those Americans who completed their studies in Scotland during the war, it was not easy to return to the States and many took jobs in Britain until the end of hostilities.

The Americans in Scotland formed American Medical Students' Clubs in both Edinburgh and Glasgow and developed the sports of baseball and American football. The American Club in Glasgow came to the attention of the local Jewish community when the Club held a dance on the eve of the Jewish Sabbath. The Americans disclaimed responsibility, being an American rather than a Jewish club. The

Glasgow *Jewish Echo* said that this was 'American humbug', as it was well known that the American medical students were almost exclusively Jewish.[33] While the relations between the Glasgow Jewish community and the American students had their ups and downs, by 1938 (when it was estimated that there were 340 in Glasgow alone), the Rev Dr IK Cosgrove, minister of the Garnethill Synagogue, said that he saw the American students as an integral part of the Jewish community.[34] In Edinburgh Rabbi Salis Daiches took an interest in the Americans and may have discussed the admission of American Jewish medical students with representatives from the University and the College of Surgeons.[35]

In 1939, when Dean Rappleye was touring Europe to inspect medical institutions where Americans were studying, there was some resentment in Edinburgh that Scottish medical organisations were being dragged into internal American medical politics. Dr John Orr, Dean of the medical school of the Royal Colleges, made it clear, in a letter to the American Students' Medical Club in Glasgow, that he regarded the inspection of his school, which had lasted only one hour, as 'very sinister'. He considered that racial discrimination entered largely into the question. He could hardly believe otherwise with a large American student body which was almost exclusively Jewish. In fact, in 1937-8 it was estimated that 90% of Americans studying medicine abroad were Jewish.[36]

The medical school of the Royal Colleges of Edinburgh also referred to the 'racial question as affecting the Jewish race' in their comments on the Goodenough Commission on Medical Education, which recommended the closure of the extra-mural schools after the war.[37] They rebutted the claims made about the American students, namely that they had been excluded from places in the United States in an attempt to improve standards. Dean Orr was aware of developments in America after his visits to universities there in 1930 and 1931. He rejected the view that the Colleges were providing a 'Scottish backdoor to the medical profession in the United States'. The records of the graduates of the extra-mural schools in the New York State Board Examinations showed the level of their ability and their training.

The English medical schools appear to have taken firmer action to enforce the suggestions of the GMC that caution be exercised in the admission of Americans. Following correspondence with the GMC in 1930, Leeds University decided not to admit American medical students. Liverpool University admitted only one American undergraduate to the Medical Faculty during the 1930s. In London, a few Americans were admitted to St Bartholomew's, King's College, and Charing Cross and Westminster. This last school currently admitted many students from countries such as India, Egypt and South Africa. It may have seemed more prudent to continue admitting students from these traditional overseas countries rather than get involved in medico-political arguments over the admission of Americans.

By comparison, the Scottish medical schools, particularly the extra-mural colleges and to a lesser extent the universities, demonstrated a combination of practical sympathy and traditional entrepreneurial skill. The extra-mural schools benefited from the influx of Americans and increased their rolls quite substantially. This was sufficient to put Scotland on the map as the major overseas centre for the training of American-born physicians during the 1930s.

The Americans undoubtedly enjoyed their years in Scotland and gained much from their Scottish medical education. They were taught observation and traditional clinical skills. Some returning physicians felt that therapeutics and medical sciences were more advanced in the United States and, especially towards the end of the 1930s, it was difficult for some returning Americans to enter appropriate intern jobs. However, many of the Scots-trained American physicians reached the top of their profession, although a relatively high number entered general practice. The Triple Qualification Board, and through them the extra-mural schools, proved to be the major beneficiaries of the events of the 1930s. As David Hamilton has written of their post-war move into post-graduate medical education, 'Adam Smith would have been proud of them!'[38]

Acknowledgements

I would like to acknowledge assistance from Dr R Smart, Keeper of the Muniments, University of St Andrews; Dr Derek Dow, Archivist, Greater Glasgow Health Board; the late Miss Dorothy Wardle, Librarian of the Royal College of Surgeons, Edinburgh; Dr JL Potter, Executive Dean of the Faculty of Medicine, University of Edinburgh; Dr Nathan Kaganoff, Librarian of the American Jewish Historical Society, Brandeis University, Waltham, Mass.; Library of the Royal College of Physicians and Surgeons of Glasgow; Colin MacLaren, Archivist, University of Aberdeen; AR Allan, Assistant Archivist, University of Liverpool. I should also like to acknowledge financial support from the Carnegie Trust for the Universities of Scotland for

a visit to New York in Spring 1986 and to the Wellcome Trust for
a grant towards a visit to Boston and Washington.

The Scottish Colleges – Teaching and Examining Abroad

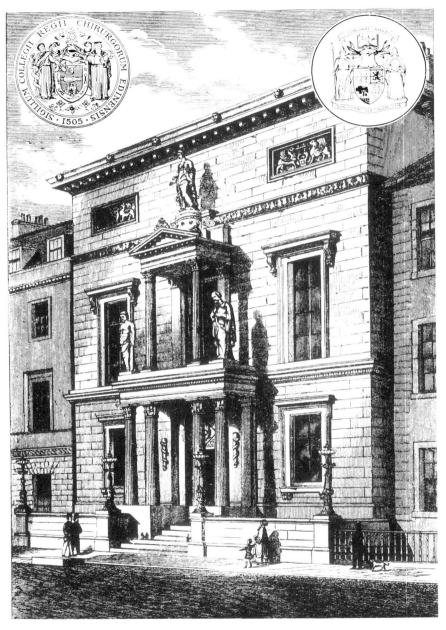

Portals of a profession. The entrance to the Royal College of Physicians of Edinburgh, flanked by the seals of the Royal College of Surgeons of Edinburgh and the Royal College of Physicians and Surgeons of Glasgow.

Chapter 12
The Scottish Colleges —
Teaching and Examining Abroad

T J Thomson

The Royal Medical Colleges in Scotland are three in number — the Royal College of Surgeons of Edinburgh (1505), the Royal College of Physicians and Surgeons of Glasgow (1599) and the Royal College of Physicians of Edinburgh (1681). This account of their overseas impact in recent years will be conducted under six separate headings — background, examinations abroad, teaching abroad, joint conferences, double sponsorship and the 'Oman Project'.

The present-day position has resulted from the activities of Scottish doctors in the past — with their tradition of pioneering abroad. Such individuals have not only gone as College representatives, but also from universities and in response to personal invitations from colleagues overseas. It would be quite impossible for me to name all of these pioneers in this field, but one of the first was Sir JDS Cameron, Past President of the RCPEd, who retired voluntarily in order to go to Dacca where he guided the development of postgraduate medical education between 1965 and 1967, setting up the Institute for Postgraduate Medicine and Research, which is still active today. This Institute has been visited subsequently by Presidents of the Royal College of Physicians of Edinburgh. The names of Professor Stanley Alstead and Professor Charles Fleming, Postgraduate Dean, come to mind in relation to the Nairobi-Makerere connection with the Glasgow medical school where members of staff at all levels were seconded to Nairobi for periods of at least one year. This began more than twenty years ago and led at that time to the appointment of three substantive professors in the University there. (Now in 1986 we have two elective students from Nairobi in our unit in Stobhill Hospital in

Glasgow. This is but one example of the unforeseen effects of a project launched many years previously).

More recently, Professor John Gillingham (Past President of the RCSEd) has led the development of neuro-surgery in Riyadh in Saudi Arabia. Yet another Past President of that College, Mr James Ross, also served in Riyadh, as Professor of Anatomy.

Another factor which has played a major part in the development of the 'Overseas Connection' has been the large number of doctors from areas such as Malaysia, Asia, Africa and the Middle East who have come to Scotland for educational courses and examinations organised by the Scottish Colleges. These were the evolutionary stages. The personal two-way contacts maintained over the years between representatives of the Colleges here, and governments, universities, colleges and postgraduate institutions abroad have all strengthened the bonds between our Colleges and the educational bodies overseas.

Thus it is on this breadth of experience and on a background of mutual respect and friendship that the Scottish Colleges have in recent years been active in teaching and examining abroad.

Within the compass of this paper it is possible only to indicate some of the highlights of activity and illustrate the general philosophies in a changing field. The first area to be reviewed is that of examining abroad. The diploma examinations held overseas include the MRCP(UK) Parts I and II, the FRCS(Ed) Primary and Final, and the FRCS(Glasg) Primary and Final. The Colleges have no wish to impose the examinations and only agree to hold them abroad when a formal request is received from the country concerned. The MRCP(UK) exams are of course organised jointly with the Royal College of Physicians of London. It is worth noting that the Part I consists only of a multiple choice question paper.

The MRCP(UK) Part I is currently (1986) held in fourteen countries. (Abu Dhabi, Egypt, Ghana, Hong Kong, Iraq, Jordan, Kuwait, Malaysia, Oman, Saudi Arabia, Sri Lanka, Sudan, West Indies, Zimbabwe). It all began in Sri Lanka in 1971 and the most recent centre to be involved is Oman, where it was planned for July of this year. It was also held in Iran for six years and on one occasion in Ethiopia. The examination is held three times a year at the same hour on the same day in all centres throughout the world. In some instances, these countries serve as regional centres, with candidates travelling from adjacent countries to sit the examination.

There are many advantages to the host country in having such examinations there. They stimulate interest and activity in postgraduate medical education locally and, indeed, we have seen the development of courses parallel the holding of exams. Furthermore, the doctors can sit the examination whilst continuing to practise in their own Health Services, avoiding the need to travel to the UK with the attendant financial outlays and separation from families. Increasing familiarity with the format of the exam has led colleges and postgraduate institutes overseas to introduce similar examinations for their own diplomas, a theme which will be developed in a later section of this paper.

The MRCP(UK) Part II follows a well established format incorporating written, clinical and oral sections, a structure which raises some problems in any proposal to export this part of the examination. The written papers are based on projected slide material as well as clinical problems in printed book form. There then follow in about four weeks the clinical and oral sections of the exam. To maintain the same standard in all centres, even in the UK, the projection facilities must be virtually identical. To ensure this overseas could prove difficult but the Joint Examining Board of the Colleges of Physicians of the UK is looking at this problem, and, indeed, in October 1985 the total Part II Examination was held in Hong Kong and it is planned to have the written part of the exam in Malaysia this year. A news release from the University of Hong Kong at the time of the exam emphasised the importance of this development:

> 'This is a landmark in the history of local postgraduate medical education and an important catalyst to Hong Kong's postgraduate medical training'.

If we look now at the examinations of the Surgical Colleges we find the Edinburgh College of Surgeons conducts these in Hong Kong, Kuala Lumpur, Riyadh and Singapore and the Glasgow College in Kuwait, Abu Dhabi and formerly in Tripoli. The FRCS exam involves orals in both Primary and Final sections so that teams of College examiners, including external examiners, must attend at each examination centre.

It is important to realise that many countries have acquired their own postgraduate diplomas over the last ten to fifteen years, and the following qualifications now gain exemption from the Primary FRCS in Scotland: MMed Singapore, MMed Nairobi, DM West Indies, MCS Sudan, MS Sri Lanka, MMed Makerere (prior to 1972), MMed Nigeria (now known as the Fellowship of the Nigerian Medical Council),

Fellowship of the West African College of Surgeons (when candidate has passed the Primary and Part I of the Final). In addition, there is reciprocity and exemption with the Primary from the Royal College of Surgeons in Ireland, the RCS of England, the Royal Australasian College of Surgeons and the College of Physicians, Surgeons and Gynaecologists of South Africa.

This again, like the MRCP(UK) Part I, has the benefit of allowing in-service training at home in these countries and their examinations take account of national requirements and local needs.

Perhaps at this stage I can summarise some of the general points which we have learned in relation to the examinations abroad:

a)   Training is more important than the examination.

b)   The use made of the exam will vary in different countries. Ireland uses the Part I MRCP(UK) on an agency basis and validated questions from the banks of questions are being used as sections of diploma exams in countries abroad, e.g. in Sri Lanka as part of its Part I Examination, with added questions related to local needs; validated material is incorporated locally, e.g. in the MMed of Sudan.

c)   The common aim is for countries abroad to develop their own first postgraduate diplomas, relevant to their own national requirements. This change has occurred in a prospective fashion in recent years. As a result, representatives from Colleges are being invited to advise on training methods and standards of examinations in several countries; I myself examined in the College of West Africa in Ibadan, as have several Presidents of the RCPEd, while Professor John Strong of Edinburgh and I acted together as external examiners in the College of Physicians and Surgeons of Pakistan in Karachi. This is a developing process, the rate of progress varying from country to country.

If we turn now to formalised teaching by the Colleges in overseas countries, this is much less clearly defined. Again, as with examinations, this only occurs in response to formal requests from the countries concerned. Every second year the Royal College of Surgeons of Edinburgh sends a team of lecturers in the basic sciences to Kuala Lumpur. The Glasgow College formerly organised in Tripoli a course for the Primary FRCS with some participation from local teachers, but this has not been held in recent years. In Kuwait, assistance is given when requested in courses arranged locally. All three Colleges participate in teaching abroad, through individuals invited to lecture formally or to teach at the bedside or in clinical seminars. These invitations often arise from personal contacts which are made by meeting with colleagues from abroad, at conferences or at representative meetings.

It may appear that the arrangements for examinations abroad and the sharing of educational expertise have arisen in a somewhat *ad hoc* fashion, but this is not entirely so. While there will always be advancing thrusts by individuals in any joint enterprise, the Colleges here and the medical institutions abroad have held International Conferences to discuss the standards of training and examining and plans for postgraduate medical education.

On the surgical side there is a joint Conference of Surgical Colleges founded in 1970 with membership from former Commonwealth countries. This now meets overseas in alternate years. Themes regularly discussed include the possible reciprocity of College exams and the development of diplomas of comparable high standards (both of which have been mentioned previously), the exchange of external examiners and the introduction of exchange travelling fellowships.

The exchange of examiners is occurring between the countries overseas as well as with ourselves in this country. Exchange travelling fellowships are attractive in theory, but the practical difficulties can be considerable. Ideally, there would be an exchange of doctors in similar posts at similar stages of training in each of the two countries. They could simply transfer to each other's posts and (possibly) domiciles, the service work of the units continuing much as before. With few exceptions, this has proved difficult to implement for a variety of reasons. These include the problem of identifying people who are appropriate for such a scheme and who are prepared to commit themselves for a specific period. Financial implications may also be a drawback, as can inability to benefit from the environment while living away from home and family. The principle is an excellent one, however, and individual cases can be very successful. There has recently been an exchange in the specialty of orthopaedics, wherein an established doctor from Oman has received higher surgical training in Scotland, while at the same time senior registrars in that specialty have been seconded from Glasgow and Edinburgh for periods of six months or so to Oman.

Within the past decade the Colleges of Physicians of the United

Kingdom have organised two major conferences with colleagues from overseas. Held in 1977 and 1983, these are now referred to as the 'Leeds Castle Conferences'. A number of the themes discussed at these meetings have had a considerable influence on present-day practices. The 1977 Conference, attended by representatives of seven overseas countries (Egypt, Ghana, Malaysia, Nigeria, Sri Lanka, Sudan and the West Indies) produced several major recommendations. Two of these — the exchange of examiners and a proposal to hold a workshop on examination overseas — have already been adopted. The provision of approved posts in the UK proved to be impractical. Under this proposal it was suggested that some substantive posts might be reserved by government, training committees or Colleges for doctors from overseas. However, with the strong competition for such posts in this country following on open advertisement, it had to be pointed out that no institution had the authority to reserve posts. In short, this was not an acceptable proposition, but it is interesting to find more recently, under what is termed a 'Double Sponsorship Scheme', that doctors from overseas are, indeed, working in approved training posts in the NHS.

As regards recognition of the work of UK doctors overseas, this has also been a 'late developer'. Only in the last few years has formal recognition and approval been given in selected instances for doctors from Glasgow and Edinburgh to work in Oman for limited periods.

My own notes after attending the 1977 Conference record that at that time I felt that education was required to ensure that governments and ministries abroad understood that the UK Colleges considered the membership examination to be an indication of suitability for further training and not as an exit exam indicating a trained specialist. Indeed, it was clear even then, in discussion with colleagues from abroad, that our Colleges could make a major contribution in post-diploma training for what has now come to be known as higher specialist training.

By the time of the second Conference in 1983 some of the 1977 recommendations had been achieved, but further developments were recognised as desirable. Many countries were organising postgraduate courses and there was a great need for teachers from the UK to assist in these. Such visits could be short-term or long-term, depending on the circumstances. In the latter case thought was given to the recruitment of retired consultants. Again, reference was made to test material. The concepts of dual sponsorship and recognition of post-diploma training were formally recognised at that time.

There are two levels at which doctors from abroad may take postgraduate training. The first is at the stage of general professional training leading ordinarily to the FRCS or MRCP(UK) diplomas. The second is at the post-diploma stage. There are two important features of this whole concept which must be kept in mind. It is likely that with the increase in the number of national diplomas abroad, the number of young doctors coming to the UK at the pre-diploma stage in their careers will fall over the next few years, while in the present climate it is very unlikely that any doctor coming to this country without double sponsorship will obtain a satisfactory training post.

The College in Glasgow has had a dual sponsorship scheme since 1982. This followed on discussions with senior colleagues abroad who welcomed the proposal that the College should supervise the training of selected doctors coming to the West of Scotland. The principles which guide this scheme are as follows. The doctor must have passed the Primary FRCS or MRCP(UK) Part I examination, or one of equivalent status. Requests for training are made by the government or a national institution of the country concerned, but not by an individual. The same authority sponsors the candidate financially (one part of the double sponsorship, the second being the role of the College). The doctor will have had at least one year's experience in the subject in his own country and the English linguistic ability must be certified. Wherever practical, any candidate for the scheme is interviewed by a representative of the College before acceptance. The College, through its Overseas Committee, has identified suitable training posts in hospitals in the West of Scotland, with the willing agreement of the nominated trainers who are consultants in these hospitals. Application is made by the College to the General Medical Council for limited registration in relation to the individual doctor and a particular post. This allows exemption from the Professional and Linguistics Asessments Board (PLAB) test. When this Limited Registration (LR) is obtained the doctor is offered a substantive unfunded post in which he is an active member of the unit. The level of responsibility which he can assume is assessed after the first three months. Each doctor is interviewed at the College soon after taking up post and at intervals of six to nine months thereafter. Confidential reports on progress are submitted by the consultant to the College. If the individual trainee is not working satisfactorily, the double sponsorship is withdrawn and the candidate is requested to return to his own country.

The second element of the scheme concerns training in the post-diploma stage. It is very clear in personal meetings, both with university and ministry colleagues abroad, that they would wish selected doctors to have supervised higher specialist training in this country in order that they can be appointed to senior posts on their return home. Candidates are required to have passed the examination at the end of general professional training, the FRCS or MRCP(UK) or equivalent, and the College prepares the way by arranging such matters as limited registration from GMC. There are unfunded senior registrar posts in this country which have been approved by the relevant Higher Training Committees. These are suitable for use in the double sponsorship scheme, and, indeed, some of them are being used at the present time. The College supervision is as previously described, and the duration can vary from three months to four years. Discussions are currently in progress about the award of a certificate in recognition of the supervised training in the specialty which the doctor receives under the scheme.

The development of the Glasgow College Scheme (for which no fees are levied) has involved considerable activity overseas, advising on training and on the approval of posts in the countries to which it has been extended. By July 1986 the scheme involved Trainees from Jordan, Kuwait, Libya, Oman, Malaysia and Turkey. Of the twenty-four who had completed their course or were currently in training, no fewer than eleven came from Oman, with a further seven from Libya. Another seven had been accepted for training, but had not yet taken up post. Specialist training has been offered in no fewer than nine separate fields: paediatrics; general and cardiothoracic surgery; surgical urology; gastroenterology; respiratory medicine; nephrology; communicable diseases; clinical immunology.

The concluding section of this paper focusses on a further and important collaborative venture by the Glasgow College, in what I have called 'The Oman Project'. This is yet another example of developments which can result from personal contacts made many years previously. A Fellow of the Glasgow College had been in Oman during his national service, making friends and medical contacts in that country. Later, as a consultant in orthopaedic surgery, he was instrumental in initiating the exchange scheme in the specialty of orthopaedics to which I referred earlier.

It was against this background that the Minister of Health in Oman visited the Glasgow College in 1983 to discuss how collaboration with the College might further the development of medical services and education in Oman. The first fruits of these discussions resulted in the appointment of a Director of Laboratory Services in 1984. Since then many medical laboratory scientific officers in various laboratory disciplines have gone on unpaid leave to work in Oman. These scientific officers are working with personnel in the Health Service there and are playing an active part in the development of the laboratory services. There is now a reciprocal movement, with scientific officers and doctors from Oman gaining experience in laboratories in Glasgow, under the Double Sponsorship Scheme. As in so many other enterprises the College does not work alone in this venture, but is dependent upon the close collaboration of both the University of Glasgow and the Greater Glasgow Health Board.

As regards surgery, a Director was appointed in April 1985 and regular postgraduate medical educational meetings are taking place. In anaesthetics, the appointment of two successive senior registrars from Glasgow has given continuity of services in Oman and there have been short-term visits from consultants in that specialty. Advice has been given in relation to radiological services and a Director in this specialty took up post in 1985; he was preceded by a senior radiographer in 1984.

A subsequent offshoot of such joint enterprises has been the secondment of several fully trained nurses to Oman, the result of a request by the Omani Minister of Health to the Greater Glasgow Health Board.

I have been privileged to be associated with the Oman Project since its inception in 1983, serving as a member of the Postgraduate Medical Education Committee. Seminars and clinical meetings are held in many hospitals throughout the country. Symposia are arranged, at least one major one annually, with participants from all parts of Oman. The first of these, held in 1984, was an international symposium on gastroenterology, organised jointly by the Postgraduate Committee and the Glasgow College. Speakers came from Kuwait, Glasgow and Oman and some 250 delegates attended. A second joint symposium on cardio-vascular subjects is planned for the future. The Oman Project represents a natural development in the role of Colleges, sharing the benefits of our experiences with colleagues overseas.

The Postgraduate Medical Education Committee has supervised the development of the *Oman Medical Newsletter*, a quarterly production which celebrated its second anniversary in August 1986. The articles relate to medical practice in Oman. It may well be that this will become their national medical journal.

Within the context of this necessarily brief paper, I have offered a glimpse of the origins, subsequent developments and future aspirations of the Scottish Royal Colleges in teaching and examining abroad. I am sure we would all agree with the view endorsed by the Presidents of the Colleges of Physicians in the United Kingdom after the Leeds Castle Conference of 1983:

> 'that medical problems must be considered on an international basis, and friendship between physicians (and surgeons) is one of the best ways of promoting the advancement of knowledge, co-operation in research, the improvement of medical care and understanding between nations'.

Finally, this work abroad cannot be done without Scottish expatriates working in these countries. WS Craig's *History of the Royal College of Physicians of Edinburgh*, published in 1976, suggests that we should all spare a thought for such expatriates, expressing the sentiment which inspired Charles Murray to write:

> 'Here on the Rand we freely grant
> We're blest wi' sunny weather;
> Fae cauld an' snaw we're weel awa',
> But man, we miss the heather.'

Notes

Introduction
D A Dow

1. Comrie, J.D., *History of Scottish Medicine* (London 1932), Vol. II, 715-86. David Hamilton's more recent work, *The Healers: A History of Scottish Medicine* (Edinburgh 1981) contains passing references to the influence of Scots outwith Scotland, but only in very general terms.

2. Brown, P.H., *A Short History of Scotland* (Edinburgh 1908), new edition revised by H.W. Meikle (1955), 324.

3. Burton, J.H., *The Scot Abroad* (Edinburgh 1881), *passim*.

4. Lenman, Bruce, *Integration, Enlightenment and Industrialization. Scotland 1746-1832* (London 1981), 92. See also Cage, R.A., 'The Scots in England' in Cage, R.A. (ed.), *The Scots Abroad. Labour, Capital, Enterprise, 1750-1914* (London 1985), 43, where the author describes the pioneering work of Hunter and Smellie in *surgery*.

5. See, for example, Brown, *op. cit.*, 326; Donaldson, G., *The Scots Overseas* (London 1966), 182-3; Checkland, Sydney and Checkland, Olive, *Industry and Ethos. Scotland 1832-1914* (London 1984), 161.

6. Lenman, *op. cit.*, 80ff.

7. Harvie, Christopher, *No Gods and Precious Few Heroes. Scotland 1914-1980* (London 1981), *passim*. Christopher Smout's *A Century of the Scottish People 1830-1950* (London 1986) is equally uninformative.

8. Aspinwall, B., 'The Scots in the United States' in Cage, *op. cit.*, 86.

9.   See Appleby, J.H., 'Through the Looking-Glass: Scottish Doctors in Russia (1704-1854)' in *The Caledonian Phalanx. Scots in Russia* (National Library of Scotland 1987), 47-60; Appleby, J.H., 'British Doctors in Russia 1657-1807' (East Anglia PhD 1979); Ashbee, F., 'George Lyon Carrick, Scots Physician in Tsarist Russia' in *Scottish Slavonic Review* (1983), *I*, 73-84.

10. Christie, D., *Ten Years in Manchuria. A Story of Medical Mission Work in Moukden 1883-1893* (Paisley n.d.), *passim*. Christie, Mrs. D., *Dugald Christie of Manchuria. Pioneer and Medical Missionary* (London 1932), *passim;* Hewat, E.G.K., *Vision and Achievement 1796-1956. A History of the Foreign Missions of the Churches United in the Church of Scotland* (London 1960), 263.

11. Hargreaves, J.D., *Aberdeenshire to Africa. Northeast Scots and British Overseas Expansion* (Aberdeen 1981), 72-3.

12. See, for example, a series of articles on Henry Faulds (in Japanese with English abstracts) by Nagatoya, Y., in *Jou. Nissei Hosp.* (1974), *2,* 137–41; (1976), *4(1),* 131–8; (1977), *5(1),* 141–7.

13. Cortazzi, H., *Dr. Willis in Japan 1862-1877. A British medical pioneer* (London 1985); obituary notice of Willis in *Brit. Med. Jou.* (24 February 1894), 441.

14. Hargreaves, *op. cit.*, 73.

15. Senex, *Glasgow Past and Present* (Glasgow 1884), *Vol. III*, 500-1.

16. Dr David Coats was the brother of James and Peter Coats, joint founders of the famous Paisley thread firm of J. & P. Coats Ltd. He joined the practice in Rio de Janeiro of his second cousin, Dr Henry Coats. David's health failed after two years and he died in America in 1856. See Coates, A., *From The Cottage to The Castle* (privately printed 1894), 49-52.

The Medical Traffic with Europe

J D Galbraith.

1.   'The Middle Ages' has for long been an accepted, if imprecise, term (?the middle of what?) and since it becomes particularly inconvenient at both ends, whenever they were, it is only fair to

point out that this paper has been confined to the period between A.D. 563 (Columba's landing on Iona, according to Adomnan) and 1513 (James IV's defeat at Flodden).

2. This belief has been remarkably durable, even though Merton College was evidently teaching, and awarding degrees in medicine from the early part of the 14th century, at least. For a discussion of the faculty of medicine at Aberdeen which puts it in proper perspective, see Macfarlane, L.J., *William Elphinstone and the Kingdom of Scotland, 1431-1514* (Aberdeen 1985), 322-3, 382-5.

3. The fact that Elphinstone had 'gaderit' these legends is expressed in the patent granted, in 1507, to Walter Chapman and Andrew Millar, Scotland's first printers. See Livingstone, M. (ed.), *Registrum Secreti Sigilli Regum Scotorum* (Edinburgh 1908), *I*, No.1546. The national 'propaganda' in the resulting compilation, (*Breviarii Aberdonensis ad percelebris ecclesie Scotorum potissimum usum et consuetudinem*, Edinburgh, 1510, which title rather speaks for itself) is so pervasive as to defeat specific citation here.

4. Myln, Alexander, 'Vitae Episcoporum Dunkeldense' in Hannay, R.K. (ed.), *Rentale Dunkeldense* (Edinburgh 1915), 313.

5. Macfarlane, *op.cit.*, 385.

6. Anderson, A.O. and Anderson, M.O., *Adomnan's Life of Columba* (Edinburgh 1961), 364.

7. Mackinlay, J.M., *Ancient Church Dedications* (Edinburgh 1914) II, 50; and, for example, Maclean, G.R.D. (ed.), *Poems of the Western Highlanders* (London 1961), 206-7. For the reputation of the 'moderworth' elsewhere in these islands, see Bonser, Wilfred, *The Medical Background of Anglo-Saxon England* (London 1963), 335-6. The association with St John is worth a passing mention, since it was to this evangelist, according to the testimony of St Colman at the Synod of Whitby (at any rate, as reported by Bede) that the 'Celtic' church owed its distinctive customs.

8. Cockayne, Revd Oswald (ed.), *Leechdoms, Wortcunning and Starcraft of Early England . . .* i.e. Thomas Oswald, in *Rerum Brittanicum Medii Aevi Scriptores* (London 1864-6), *II*, 113-5, 157.

9. In the Highlands, Columba was a protector of cattle: in (the

presumably more rural) Germany, he was a protector of fields.
See Bonser, *op. cit.*, 437.

10.   *Breviarium Practice*, bk. 3, cap. 17, in Arnaldi de Villanova . . .
      Opera nuperrime revisa (imp. Guilelmus Huyon, Lyon, 1520). The
      invocation of St Brandan (?*recte* St Patrick) appears on fo. 192v
      of this edition, which is cited hereafter as Arnaldus, *Breviarium*.

11.   Probably the best account, still, of the Irish scholars in Europe
      is in Waddell, Helen, *The Wandering Scholars* (London 1927),
      Chapter 2, part II onwards.

12.   See, for example, Haskins, C.H., *The Rise of Universities* (New
      York 1940), 8-9; for the participation of Scots in the Crusades,
      see Macquarrie, Alan, *Scotland and the Crusades, 1095-1560*
      (Edinburgh 1985).

13.   Thorndike, Lynn, *Michael Scot* (London 1965), 11.

14.   The evidence, which is presumptive rather than definite, is
      discussed in Thorndike, *op. cit.*, 11-2, Haskins, C.H., *Studies in the
      History of Medieval Science* (New York 1960), 272-3, and Watt,
      D.E.R., *Biographical Dictionary of Scottish Graduates to 1410* (Oxford
      1977), 490. Michael seems never to have been claimed by the
      Irish, unlike the theologian John Duns Scotus, but in Michael's
      case this is perhaps not too suprising.

15.   A Sir Michael Scott of Balwearie appears in various records
      between 1290 and 1310, which, as the scholar died around 1236,
      was evidently close enough for Sir Walter to make the
      connection, if it had not already been made for him by Hector
      Boece. The contrast with Bacon (who cheated by using a magic
      lantern) is in Hogg's *Three Perils of Man* (1822), chapter 15.

16.   From a sermon preached by Helinand of Froidmont (?d. 1772) at
      Toulouse, in Minge, J.P. (ed.), *Patrologiae Cursus Completus* etc.,
      [*Patrologiae Latina*], (Paris 1855), *vol. 212*, column 603. 'They [the
      scholars] seek knowledge everywhere, but life nowhere' he
      gloomily adds.

17.   Thorndike, *op. cit.*, 32.

18.   Holder-Egger, C. (ed.), *Cronica Fratris Salimbene de Adam ordinus
      Minorum a 1250*, in *Monumenta Germaniae Historica Scriptorum*

(Hanover 1905-13), *vol. 32*, 349; 'I . . . once loved him, for he wrote for me to Brother Elias, minister-general of the Franciscans, that . . . he might restore me to my father'. Whatever his merits as a chronicler, Salimbene [hereafter cited as such] is at his best as a raconteur *cum* moralist. His final verdict on Frederick is 'A little rotteness destroys the whole apple'.

19. Salimbene, 174.

20. Walter Scott, 'The Lay of the Last Minstrel', canto II, xiii
              '. . . when in Salamanca's cave
              Him listed his magic wand to wave
              The bells would ring in Notre Dame'.

21. Dante, 'L'Inferno', canto xx.

22. Salimbene, 512.

23. Denifle, H. and Chatelain, A. (eds.), *Chartularium Universitatis Parisiensis* (Paris 1889), *vol. I*, 105, 110.

24. Salimbene, 353. Scott himself seemingly said that the building was a church tower; see Thorndike, *op. cit.*, 19, 45.

25. *Compendium Studii Philosophae*, in Brewer, J.S. (ed.), *Fr Rogeri Bacon Opera . . . Inedita*.

26. Haskins, *Studies*, 279.

27. Thorndike, *op. cit.*, 25.

28. Arnaldus, *Breviarium*, bk. 4, cap. 10 (fos. 198-198v in the edition of 1520). Thorndike, *op. cit.*, 72 quotes De Renzi, *Collectio Salernitana*, (1852), I, 292 to the effect that the *Breviarium* 'frequently cites' Michael Scot, but points out that such citation was not noticable in the edition he consulted; this is the only such instance I have found.

29. The treatise is discussed in Haskins, *Studies*, 299-326.

30. Salimbene, 350, 353.

31. Thorndike, *op. cit.*, 72-3.

32. *ibid.*, 76; Haskins, *Studies*, 289 n.108.

33. For these inhaled narcotics, see Thorndike, L., *Science and Thought in the Fifteenth Century* (New York 1929), 5.

34. Thorndike, *Scot*, 74.

35. For a discussion of Michael's medical knowledge, see Thorndike, *Scot*, 72-8.

36. Bacon, Roger, *De erroribus medicorum*, trans. E.T. Withington, in Singer, Charles and Sigerist, H.E. (eds.), *Essays on the History of Medicine presented to Karl Sudhoff* (Oxford and Zurich 1924), 144.

37. Wickersheimer, Ernest, *Dictionnaire Biographique des Medecins en France au Moyen Age* (Paris 1936). 75, seems prepared to accept Bernard's Scottish origins on the sole grounds that Chaucer couples his name with those of John of Gaddesden and Gilbertus Anglicus, who were English (Prologue to 'The Canterbury Tales', line 434).

38. Dunlop, A.I., *Scots Abroad in the Fifteenth Century* (Historical Association 1942), 17.

39. As says Bernard Gordon in his *proemium* to *Lilium Medicinae*, citing Socrates, Horace and Seneca in support. But this was not entirely so, even in Bernard's day, for by the later 13th century some universities, notably Paris, had begun to regulate their book-sellers, and to make, *inter alia*, provision for the hiring out of parts (*pecia*) of standard texts which had been certified correct, for copying by students and scribes. Surviving pecia are mostly of texts required for the study of theology and the laws the best-known list of what texts were available (Paris, ?1275) apparently includes no medical works at all. See Denifle and Chatelaine, *op.cit.*, 644-9. However, the system did extend to the study of medicine also. Jean Destrez in the standard work on the subject, points out that the Bologna statutes of 1405 contain a list of 23 medical works, and that Bernard's *Lilium* may have been copied at Paris; see Destrez, *La Pecia dans les manuscrits Universitaires du XIIIe et XIVe siecle* (Paris 1935), 32, 95 and plates 14-5. The application of the 'pecia system' to medicine would be well worth further study.

40. The teaching of medicine is discussed in detail by Talbot, Charles, 'Medical Education in the Middle Ages' in O'Malley, C.D. (ed.), *The History of Medical Education* (Berkeley 1970), 73-87, from which most of what follows has been developed.

41. *ibid.*, 80.

42. The distinction between 'phisicius' (a philosophical physician) and the mere 'mercenary healing of bodies' (*ibid.*, 83) which was the province of the 'medicus' does not seem to have been particularly clear in Scotland.

43. Canon 10; Mansi, J.D. (ed.), *Sacrorum Conciliorum Nova et Amplissima Collectio . . .* (Venice 1778), 22, 998-9, and Alberigo, J. *et al.* (eds.), *Conciliorum Oecumenicorum Decreta* (Freiburg 1962), 215-6.

44. For example, see Banks, M.M. (ed.), *Alphabetum Narrationum* of Etienne de Besancon (London 1904).

45. Though Guy de Chauliac was less than complimentary on the subject of the *Rosa Anglica seu Rosa Medicinae* of John of Gaddesden (c.1280-1349), Chaucer seems to have regarded its author as one of the greatest authorities of his day (note 37 above). It is reported by the Rev. Donald Macqueen of Kilmuir that Fearcher Beaton (? died c.1596) so valued his Gaelic translation of Bernard's *Lilium* that he would send it by land whenever he took boat for Dunvegan. (Note of 5 May 1784 in the edition of the *Lilium* printed at Lyon in 1574, held by the National Library of Scotland, and see Bannerman, John, *The Beatons* (Edinburgh 1986), 56-7). See also Talbot, C.H. and Hammond, E.A., *The Medical Practitioners in Medieval England* (London 1965), 148-50.

46. Arnaldus, *Breviarium*, bk. 4, cap. 11 (folios 199, 203v. in the edition of 1520).

47. Thorndike, *Science*, 22.

48. Mansi, *op. cit.*, 22, 1007; Alberigo *et al.*, *op.cit.*, 220.

49. Talbot, Charles, *op. cit.*, 80-2.

50. *ibid.*, 81.

51. For example, Thorndike, *Science*, chapter 2, on 'Medicine versus Law at Florence', 24-58.

52. Haskins, *Studies*, 15.

53. Dunlop, *op. cit.*, 14.

54. Cameron, A.I. (A.I. Dunlop), 'Scottish students at Paris University, 1466-1492' in *Juridical Review* (1936), xlviii, 247-8.

George Hepburn, bachelor of St Andrews, explained to the German nation at Paris that he had been unable to present himself because of pirates and other hindrances at sea.

55.   Dunlop, *op. cit.*, 18.

56.   Watt, D.E.R., 'Scottish student life abroad in the fourteenth century', in *Scottish Historical Review* (1980) *59*, 18-9.

57.   *ibid.*, 19.

58.   *Liber Procuratorum Nationis Anglicanae (Alemanniae)*, in Denifle, H. and Chatelaine, A. (eds.), *Universitate Parisiensi . . . 1406-1466* (Paris 1937), (*Auctarium Chartularii Universitatis Parisiensis*, bk. II, 615, note 3).

59.   Watt, D.E.R., 'Scottish University Men of the Thirteenth and Fourteenth Centuries' in Smout, T.C. (ed.), *Scotland and Europe 1200-1850* (Edinburgh 1986), 12.

60.   From the *Practica* of Joannes Arculanus (Venice 1493), quoted in Talbot, Charles, *op.cit.*, 84.

61.   Wulff, Winifred (ed.), *Rosa Anglica seu Rosa Medicinae . . .* of John of Gaddesden (London 1929), 291.

62.   Prologue to 'The Canterbury Tales', lines 441-4.

63.   Talbot and Hammond, *op.cit.*, 35, concerning the case of Denis Cacherna of Ireland, deprived of his canonry in 1400 for this reason.

64.   The quotation is from the 'Declaration of Arbroath' of 1320.

65.   The medical books of William Schevez are described in J.D. Comrie's chapter on the Middle Ages in *History of Scottish Medicine* (London 1932); for the medieval Gaelic manuscripts reported as having belonged to Fergus Beaton of South Uist and others of that kindred, see Bannerman, *op.cit.*, 111-9.

66.   Edict of the Diet of Worms, 7 August 1495, quoted in Sudhoff, Karl (ed.), adapted Singer, Charles, *The Earliest Printed Literature on Syphilis, being Ten Tractates from the Years 1495-1498* (Florence 1925), xix.

67.   *ibid.*, xxxix, xlv. It is perhaps worth adding that the Scottish

connection with Tubingen may have already begun; John Gray, a graduate of Cologne, was at the university there by 1500. See Dunlop, *op.cit.*, 16.

68.   *Extracts from the Council Register of the Burgh of Aberdeen, 1391-1570* (Aberdeen 1844), 425.

69.   *Extracts from the Records of the Burgh of Edinburgh, A.D. 1403-1528* (Edinburgh 1869), 71.

70.   Salimbene, 350.

71.   Mackay, A.J.G. (ed.), *The Historie and Cronicles of Scotland . . . by Robert Lindesay of Pitscottie* (Edinburgh 1899), I, 237.

The Scots and Military Medicine
J S G Blair

1.   *Textbook of Small Arms* (1929); Montgomery of Alamein, Viscount, *A History of Warfare* (London 1968).

2.   Duncan, A., *Memorials of the Faculty of Physicians and Surgeons of Glasgow, 1599-1850* (Glasgow 1896), 22-3.

3.   See Wiseman, Richard, *Eight Chirurgical Treatises* (London 1705), 4th edition. Wiseman was Sergeant Chirurgeon to King Charles II.

4.   Crawford, D.G., *History of the Indian Medical Service* (London 1914).

5.   *Records of Marischal College and the University of Aberdeen, vol. II.*

6.   McDonald, D., *Surgeons Twoe and a Barber. Being Some Account of the Life and Work of the Indian Medical Service, 1600-1947* (London 1950).

7.   Salmond, J.B., *The 51st Highland Division* (Edinburgh 1953).

8.   See obituary in Gunner (July 1979), 104; personal communication from E. Leeson.

The Influence of Scotland
on North American Medicine
R H Girdwood

Agnew, L.R.C., in O'Malley, C.D. (ed.), *The History of Medical Education* (Berkeley 1970).

Anderson, R.G.W. and Simpson, A.D.C., *The Early Years of the Edinburgh Medical School* (Edinburgh 1976).

Asimor, I., *The Birth of the United States, 1763-1816* (London 1974).

Bell, W.J., 'North American and West Indian Graduates of Glasgow and Aberdeen to 1800' in *Jou. Hist. Med.* (1965), *20*, 411-5.

Blanton, W.B., *Medicine in Virginia in the Eighteenth Century* (Richmond 1931).

Haus, C.H., *Scots in the Old Dominion, 1685-1800* (Edinburgh 1980).

McLachlan, G. (ed.), *Medical Education and Medical Care: A Scottish-American Symposium* (Oxford 1977).

Mercer, W., 'The Contribution of Edinburgh to Early American Medicine' in *Jou. Roy. Coll. Surg. Edin.* (1961), 7, 180–94.

Newman, C., *The Evolution of Medical Practice in the Nineteenth Century* (London 1957).

Riggs, A.R., 'The Colonial American Medical Student at Edinburgh' in *Univ. Edin. Jou.* (1961), *20*, 141-53.

Underwood, E.A., *Boerhaave's Men* (Edinburgh 1977).

The 250th and 100th Anniversaries of the Royal Infirmary of Edinburgh and the 100th Anniversary of the Simpson Memorial Maternity Pavilion (Edinburgh 1979).

Scottish Man-Midwives in 18th Century London
J Willocks

1. Spencer, H.R., *The History of British Midwifery from 1650 to 1800* (London 1927), 3.

2. Radcliffe, W., *Milestones in Midwifery* (Bristol 1967).

3.   Browne, O.T.D., *The Rotunda Hospital 1745-1945* (Edinburgh 1947).

4.   Glaister, J., *Dr. William Smellie and his Contemporaries* (Glasgow 1898).

5.   Willocks, J., 'William Smellie and the Birth of Modern Obstetrics' in *Surgo (1966), 33,* 4.

6.   *McLintock, A.H. (ed.), Treatise on the Theory and Practice of Midwifery* by William Smellie, 1752-4 (London 1877), *II,* 248–52, case 186.

7.   Cameron, S.J., 'William Smellie' in *Scot. Med. Jou.* (1957), *2,* 439–44.

8.   Stevens, J., *Man-Midwifery Exposed* (London 1849).

9.   Towler, J. and Bramall, J., *Midwives in History and Society* (London 1986), 104.

10. McLintock, *op.cit., I,* 430–1.

11. Johnstone, R.W., *William Smellie, the Master of British Midwifery* (Edinburgh 1952).

12. McLintock, *op.cit., III,* case 473.

13. Smellie, W., *A Set of Anatomical Tables with explanations, etc.* (London 1754).

14. Speert, H., *Obstetric and Gynaecologic Milestones* (New York 1958), 88- 93.

15. Thomas K.B., *James Douglas of the Pouch and his pupil William Hunter* (London 1964).

16. Brock, C.H., 'James Douglas of the Pouch' in *Medical History* (1964), *18,* 162.

17. Douglas J., *Douglas Figure DF 56* (?1740), *Glasgow University Library (GUL),*

18. Douglas, J., *A Description of the Peritoneum* (London 1730), 37-8.

19. Douglas, J., *Douglas Figure DF61* (?1715), *GUL.*

20. Graham, H., *Eternal Eve* (London 1950).

21. Douglas, J., *Douglas Figure DF 14* (?1730), *GUL.*

22. Pope, A., 'The Dunciad' (1727), *4*, 393-4.

23. Paget, S., *John Hunter* (London 1897).

24. Brock, C.H. (ed.), *William Hunter 1718-1783* (Glasgow 1983), edited from the Glasgow University Library copy of Simmons, S.F., *An Account of the Life and Writings of the late William Hunter*.

25. Wilson, A., 'The Varieties of Man-Midwifery' in Bynum, W.F. and Porter, R. (eds.), *William Hunter and the Eighteenth Century Medical World* (Cambridge 1985), 360.

26. Personal communication from W.R. Winterton, Middlesex Hospital Archives.

27. Dewhurst, J., *Royal Confinements* (London 1980).

28. Hunter, W., Journal of Attendance on Queen Charlotte, (*GUL*), Hunter Ms. 636 (cited hereafter as Hunter Ms.).

29. Stark, J.N., 'An Obstetric Diary of William Hunter' in *Glas. Med. Jou.* (1908), *70*, 167, 214, 338.

30. Hunter Ms. 637, Lecture Notes, vol. 3, 125 (1775).

31. Hunter, W., *Introductory Lectures* (London 1784).

32. Hunter, W., *The Anatomy of the Human Gravid Uterus* (Birmingham 1774).

33. Thornton, J.L., *Jan van Rymsdyk, Medical Artist of the Eighteenth Century* (Cambridge 1982).

34. Hunter Ms. 637, Lecture Notes, vol. 3, 162 (1775), *GUL*.

35. Marshall, A.J., *Catalogue of the Anatomical Preparations of Dr William Hunter* (Glasgow 1970).

36. Hunter Ms. 598, A Description of the Pregnant Uterus (?1783), 72, *GUL*.

38. Oppenheimer, J., *New Aspects of John and William Hunter* (London 1946).

39. Carlyle, A., *Autobiography* (Edinburgh 1860).

40. Baldwin, J., *William Hunter, Book Collector* (Glasgow 1983).

41. Durant, G.P. and Rolfe, W.D.I., 'William Hunter as Natural Historian' in *Earth Sciences History* (1984), *3*, 9-24.

42. Hunter Ms. 637, Lecture Notes, vol. 3, 121 (1775), *GUL*.

43. Denman, T., *An Introduction to the Practice of Midwifery* (London 1824), 6th edition.

44. Ramsbotham, F.H., *The Principles and Practice of Obstetric Medicine and Surgery* (London 1867), 5th edition.

The Irish Connection

P Froggatt

1. Doolin, W., *Dublin's Medical Schools; a biographical retrospect* (London 1952); Anon, 'Account of the complete school of physic in Ireland, for the instruction of students in medicine, surgery, and pharmacy' in *Edin. Med. Jou.* (1818), *14*, 662-5.

2. Kirkpatrick, T.P.C., 'The schools of medicine in Dublin in the nineteenth century' in *Brit. Med. Jou.* (1933), *II*, 109-12.

3. Brooks, E. St.J., *Sir Hans Sloane* (London 1954). Orange was the centre of the small principality of that name possessed by the later Dutch royal family until incorporated into France by Louis XIV in 1672.

4. For example, the career of Sir Jeremiah Fitzpatrick, first (and last) Inspector of Health for Land Forces in Great Britain, 1794-1802. See MacDonagh, O., *The Inspector General: Sir Jeremiah Fitzpatrick and social reform, 1783-1802* (London 1981). Fitzpatrick was born a Catholic, became an Anglican, but reverted to Catholicism after he retired from public life.

5. Chambers, G., *Faces of Change: the Belfast and Northern Ireland Chambers of Commerce and Industry, 1783-1983* (Belfast 1983), chapter 4.

6. *The Book of Trinity College, Dublin, 1591-1891* (Belfast 1892), 107-13.

7. Comrie, J.D., *History of Scottish Medicine* (London 1932), *II*, 730; see also the *Evidence, Oral and Documentary, taken before the Commissioners for Visiting the Universities of Scotland (Glasgow)*, H.C. 1837 (93) XXXVI, Appendix, Order XXXVII, 533.

8. Kirkpatrick, *op.cit.*

9. Vaughan, W.E. and Fitzpatrick, A.J. (eds.), *Irish Historical Statistics: Population 1821-1971* (Dublin 1978), 1-16.

10. Nominal lists of Edinburgh MDs distinguishing nationality were published in the *Edinburgh Medical Journal* each year. Aberdeen awarded an MD (at King's College and Marischal College) as did the University of St Andrews, but nationality of graduates is not distinguished except in the Minute Book of King's and that incompletely. See *Scottish University Commissioners*, H.C. 1837 (94) XXXVII.I and H.C. 1837 (95) XXXVIII.

11. *ibid.*

12. I am indebted to Dr Derek Dow (Archivist, Greater Glasgow Health Board) for supplying me with these and other data relating to the University of Glasgow enrolments, and to Miss Lesley De Jean (Archivist, Lothian Health Board) and her successor, Dr Christine Johnson, for data relating to the University of Edinburgh enrolments. See also *Scottish University Commissioners (Edinburgh)*, H.C. 1837 (92) XXXVI, Appendix, Order XXX, 128-9, which broadly confirms the class list above for medical students enrolled at Edinburgh University, 1811-1830.

13. Darwin, F. (ed.), *The Life and Letters of Charles Darwin including an Autobiographical Chapter* (London 1888), *I*, 36.

14. *Scottish University Commissioners (Glasgow)*, *op.cit.*, 139-140. Jeffray went on: 'But as there is a diminution of those who came to the other classes, probably it is from the pressure of the times that fewer people in Ireland can afford to send their children to a College'. I think this questionable; educational developments within Ireland, including Belfast, are probably more important.

15. Stuart, J., *Historical Memoirs of the City of Armagh* (Dublin 1900), 406, n.64.

16. Fisher, J.R. and Robb, J.H., *Royal Belfast Academical Institution.*

Centenary volume 1810-1910 (Belfast 1913); Jamieson, J., *The History of the Royal Belfast Academical Institution 1810-1960* (Belfast 1959).

17.   Anon., *Statement of the Origin and Proceedings of the Belfast Academical Institution Since its Commencement*. (Belfast: J. Smyth, 21 December 1808).

18.   Fisher and Robb, *op.cit.*, 203. Many associated with the early years of Inst supported Irish self-government, Catholic emancipation, and franchise reform, and not always under the Crown! Government therefore viewed Inst with suspicion and on occasions hostility. The accolade of 'Royal' was given in 1831 by which time most Ulster Protestants supported the Union. (See Jamieson, *op.cit.*, chapters 1-3 for a good account).

19.   Froggatt, P., 'The Foundation of the "Inst" Medical Department and its association with the Belfast Fever Hospital' in *Ulster Med. Jou.* (1976), *45*, 107-45; Froggatt, P., 'The First Medical School in Belfast, 1835-1849' in *Medical History* (1978), *22*, 237-266. Unreferenced facts in the text can be found in this and the previous article which have extensive bibliographies and lists of primary sources; Froggatt, P., 'Medicine in Ulster: the Belfast School' in O'Brien, E., Crookshank, A. and Wolstenholme, G. (eds.), *A Portrait of Irish Medicine: an Illustrated History of Medicine in Ireland* (Dublin 1983), 183-213.

20.   *Fourth Report of the Commissioners of Irish Education Inquiry*. H.C. 1826-27 (82) XIII, 157. Evidence of J.L. Drummond, 102.

21.   Froggatt, P., 'The resignation of Robert Little from the chair of midwifery at Inst' in *Ulster Med. Jou.* (1979), *48*, 19-31; Froggatt, P. and Wheeler, W.G., 'Robert Little, MA, MD, LAH, LM, Professor of Midwifery and Diseases of Women and Children, Royal Belfast Academical Institution, 1835-1840: a Biographical Note' in *Ulster Med. Jou.* (1983), *52*, 58-66.

22.   Fraser, I.F., 'Father and Son: a Tale of Two Cities, 1801-1902' in *Ulster Med. Jou.* (1968), *37*, 1-37.

23.   Graves, R.J., 'On clinical instruction: with a comparative estimate of the mode in which it is conducted in the British and continental schools' in *London Med. Gaz.* (1832), *10*, 157-65. Graves was a Trinity College Dublin medical graduate of 1818. He was

a descendant of a Cromwelliam colonel of cavalry who obtained lands in County Limerick, was highly travelled on the continent and Britain and was a superb linguist. He was appointed visiting physician to the Meath Hospital in 1821 where he at once started to revise the clinical teaching although his classic article was not published until 11 years later.

24. Graves, R.J., *A System of Clinical Medicine,* (Dublin 1843); Lawrence, C.J., 'Early Edinburgh medicine: theory and practice' in Anderson, R.G.W. and Simpson, A.D.C. (eds.), *The Early Years of the Edinburgh Medical School* (Edinburgh 1976), 81-94.

25. Anning, S.T., 'Provincial Medical Schools in the Nineteenth Century' in Poynter, F.N.L. (ed.) *The Evolution of Medical Education in Britain* (London 1966), 121-34.

26. *The Book of Trinity College, op.cit.,* 107-13.

27. Personal communication from Dr Derek Dow.

28. *Edin. Med. Jou.,* under dates.

29. Less well known is the view from Dublin put well, if satirically, by 'Erinensis' (Dr Peter Hennis Greene) who for many years contributed satirical comment on Irish medicine to Thomas Wakley's *Lancet.* He wrote in 1827 that there were two classes of student who left Ireland to graduate at Edinburgh:

> 'The first class consists of pupils who have graduated in arts and intend to become members of the College of Physicians [of Ireland] and finally Doctors of the University of Dublin; but who, wishing to anticipate the emoluments of their profession, put their half dozen of [course or class] tickets in their pockets, cross the channel, and immediately on their return commence practice which they could not have done for many years had they awaited the tardy arrival of a degree in their native University . . . pupils of the Royal College of Surgeons [in Ireland] who, for no other reason than to qualify them to meet physicians in consultation and to evade certain restrictions imposed on them by that body . . . pass over to Edinburgh [with the requisite tickets] and return with a medical degree in their pocket and their tongue in their cheek . . . The second class of pupils . . . is made up of aspiring apothecaries . . . who unable to meet the expense of a medical education in Dublin . . . embark in the desperate adventure of living on salt herrings and taking a degree at Edinburgh. These are the heroic martyrs of abstinence and study who swell up the Irish department [of Edinburgh University]. . .'

Greene's criticism appeared in *The Lancet* (1827), *I,* 335-9 under the title of 'Sketches of the Medical Profession in Ireland, No. 18: Reduction of the Present Term of Medical Graduation in the University of Dublin considered'. This is a Dublin view and hardly represents the run of Ulster Dissenters: as late as 1891, of the 128 medical students matriculated in Trinity College, less than 10 per cent were Presbyterian. See *The Book of Trinity College*, *op.cit.*, 113.

30.   Calwell, H.G. *Andrew Malcolm of Belfast, 1818-1856: Physician and Historian* (Belfast 1977).

31.   Lawrence, *op.cit.*, 81–94.

32.   Froggatt, P., 'The Distinctiveness of Belfast Medicine and its Medical School' in *Ulster Med. Jou.* (1985), *54*, 89-108.

Scottish Doctors and the English Public Health
B White

1.   Frazer, W.M., *A History of English Public Health 1834-1939* (London 1950), 85.

2.   Simon, John, *English Sanitary Institutions* (London 1897), 284.

3.   Brockington, C. Fraser, *Medical Officers of Health 1848-1855. An Essay in Local History* (London 1955), Appendix III. I am indebted to Sir Peter Froggatt for this reference.

4.   Frazer, W.M., *Duncan of Liverpool* (London 1947).

5.   White, Brenda, 'Medical Police. Politics and Police. The Fate of John Roberton' in *Medical History* (1983), *27*, 407-22.

6.   Maclagan, Douglas, 'Forensic Medicine from a Scotch Point of View' in *Brit. Med. Jou.* (1878), *II*, 233-9. The text was taken from Maclagan's address to the 1872 annual British Medical Association meeting.

7.   Simon, *op.cit.*, 266.

8.   Lectures on Medical Jurisprudence and Medical Police, delivered by W.P. Alison and taken in note form by (Sir) Thomas Watson,

Vol. I, 2-3 of unpublished 4 vol. set in library of Royal Society of Medicine.

9.   John Glaister claimed that at that time his was the only public health laboratory in Glasgow capable of the task. See Glaister, John, 'Forensic Medicine Department, University of Glasgow' in *Methods and Problems of Medical Education* (New York 1928), 9th series, 210-1.

*   Many details of professional life and qualifications have been gathered from the *Medical Directories*, the *Dictionary of National Biography, University Calendars* and other similar published sources. For further reading on specifically related material, see:

Brotherston, J.F., 'William Pulteney Alison, Scottish Pioneer of Social Medicine' in *The Medical Officer* (6 June 1958), 331-6

Pelling, Margaret, *Cholera, Fever and English Medicine* (Oxford 1978).

Rosen, George, *From Medical Police to Social Medicine. Essays on the History of Health Care* (New York 1974).

Metz, Karl H., 'Social Thought and Social Statistics in the Early Nineteenth Century' in *International Review of Social History* (1984), *XXIX*, 255-65.

The Scottish Missionary Doctor

A C Ross

1.   Gelfand, M., *Christian Doctor and Nurse* (Johannesburg 1984), chapter 1, *passim.*

2.   Aitken, R.H., *Medicine and Missions in South Africa* (Cape Town n.d.).

3.   Gelfand, *op.cit.*, 18.

4.   Williamson, J. Rutter, *The Healing of the Nation* (London 1899).

5.   Lowe, J., *Medical Missions: Their Place and Power* (London 1886), 5.

6.   McCord, J., *My Patients were Zulus* (London 1951), 95.

7.   David Livingstone to John Kirk, 18 March 1858. Cited in Foskett, R., *The Zambesi Journals and Letters of Dr John Kirk* (Edinburgh 1965), Appendix 1.

8.   Williamson, *op.cit.*, 20-1.

9.   Lowe, *op.cit.*, 29-30.

10. For further details of this extraordinary man see Shepperson, G.A. and Price, T., *Independent African* (Edinburgh 1958).

11. Shepherd, R.H.W., *A South African Medical Pioneer* (Lovedale 1952), 92.

12. Williamson, *op.cit.*, 12.

The Scottish Enlightenment and Clinical Medicine

D. Hamilton

1.   Daiches, David, *The Scottish Enlightenment* (Edinburgh 1986); Daiches, David, Jones, Peter and Jones, Jean, *A Hotbed of Genius: The Scottish Enlightenment 1730-1790* (Edinburgh 1986). See also Stott, R.M. 'The Incorporation of Surgeons and Practice in Edinburgh 1696-1755' (Edinburgh PhD 1984) and Lawrence, C.J., 'Medicine as Culture: Edinburgh and the Scottish Enlightenment' (London PhD 1984).

2.   Morrell, J.B., 'The Rise and Fall of Scottish Science' in *Times Higher Educational Supplement* (8 April 1977), 5.

3.   Hamilton, D., *The Healers: A History of Scottish Medicine* (Edinburgh 1981).

4.   Porter, Roy, 'Was there a Medical Enlightenment in Eighteenth-Century England?' in *British Journal of Eighteenth Century Studies* (1982), *5*, 49-63.

5.   Gay, P., *The Enlightenment: An Interpretation* (London 1967), *vol. 2*, 12-23.

6.   Zimmerman, Leo, 'Surgeons and the Rise of Clinical Teaching in England' in *Bulletin of the History of Medicine* (1963), *37*, 167-78.

7.   Risse, Guenter B., *Hospital Life in Enlightenment Scotland: Care and Treatment at the Royal Infirmary of Edinburgh* (Cambridge 1986).

8.   Matthias, Peter, 'Swords and Ploughshares: the Armed Forces, Medicine and Public Health in the Late Eighteenth Century' in Winter, J.M., (ed.), *War and Economic Development* (Cambridge 1975), 73-90.

A Not-so-plain Tale from the Raj: A G McKendrick, IMS

J Aitchison and G S Watson

1.   MacAlister, D., 'The Law of the Geometric Mean' in *Proc. Roy. Soc.* (1879), *29*, 367-76.

2.   McKendrick, J.G., *The Story of My Life* (Aberdeen 1919), 81, 125.

3.   McKendrick, J.G., Statement submitted to a Committee of Senate of the University of Glasgow, to consider the position of the Professor of Physiology as regards Apparatus, etc. (1878).

4.   Sharpey-Schafer, E., obituary notice of John Gray McKendrick, F.R.S. in *Proc. Roy. Soc. Edin.* (1926), *46*, 372-4.

5.   *Brit. Med. Jou.* (9 January 1892), 103.

6.   *Nature* (21 October 1909), 483.

7.   *Westbourne School for Girls. The First Hundred Years 1877-1977* (Glasgow 1977).

8.   University of Glasgow Medical Examiners' Schedule.

9.   *Brit. Med. Jou.* (30 April 1892), 928.

10. Glasgow University Magazine (1893-94), *6*, 101; (1899-1900) *12*, 211.

11. *Medical Directory* (1913), 1999.

12. *Brit. Med. Jou.* (23 February 1901), 493.

13. *The Lancet* (6 July 1901), 45.

14. *Brit. Med. Jou.* (6 July 1901), 52-3.

15. Ross, R., *Memoirs* (London 1923), 434-54.

16. Ross Archives, Letter dated 6 August 1911 from A.G. McKendrick to R. Ross.

17. Ross, *op..cit.*, 449.

18. Ross, R., 'An application of the theory of probabilities to the study of a priori pathometry I' in *Proc. Roy. Soc.* (1916), *A92*, 204-30.

19. Ross Archives, Letter dated 12 October 1901 from A.G. McKendrick to R. Ross.

20. Ross Archives, Letter dated 24 November 1908 from A.G. McKendrick to R. Ross.

21. Harvey, W.F., obituary notice of Anderson Gray McKendrick 1876-1943 in *Edin. Med. Jou.* (1943), *50*, 500-6.

22. *Brit. Med. Jou.* (10 September 1892), 598; (16 June 1900), 1504.

23. *The Lancet* (12 June 1909), 1703.

24. Harvey, W.F. and McKendrick, A.G., *The Theory and Practice of Anti-rabic Immunisation* (Scientific Memoir No. 30, Government of India 1907).

25. Lamb, G. and McKendrick, A. G., *Observations on rabies* (Scientific Memoir No. 36, Government of India 1908).

26. McDonald, D., *Surgeons Twoe and a Barber. Being Some Account of the Life and Work of the Indian Medical Service, 1600-1947* (London 1950), 215.

27. Harvey, W.F., obituary notice of Anderson Gray McKendrick, 1876-1943 in *Roy. Soc. Edin. Year Book* (1943), 23-4.

28. McKendrick, A.G., 'Chemical Dynamics of Serum Reaction' in *Proc. Roy. Soc.* (1911), *B*, 493-512.

29. Ross Archives, Letter dated 5 August 1911 from A.G. McKendrick to R. Ross.

30. Harvey, obituary notice (see note 27 above), 24.

31. Mellor, J.W., *Higher Mathematics for Students of Chemistry and Physics,* (London 1902).

32. Harvey, obituary notice (see note 27 above), 23.

33. Kennedy, C., 'The Opsonic Index' in *The British Students' Song Book* (n.d.), 64-7.

34. Greenwood, M. and White, J.D.C., 'A biometric study of phagocytosis with special reference to the "opsonic index". First memoir. On the frequency distributions of phagocytic counts' in *Biometrika* (1907), *6*, 376-401.

35. Colebrook, L., *Biographical Memoir of Almroth Edward Wright, 1861-1947* (1948).

36. Pearson, E.S., 'Karl Pearson. An appreciation of some aspects of his life and work. Part II: 1906-1937' in *Biometrika* (1937), *29*, 161-248.

37. Harvey, W.F. and McKendrick, A.G., 'The opsonic index — a medico-statistical enquiry' in *Biometrika* (1909), 7, 64-95.

38. Ross Archives, Letter dated 5 December 1912 from A.G. Mckendrick to R. Ross.

39. McKendrick, A.G., 'The Physical Aspect of the Opsonic Index' in *Science Progress 8* (1914), 497.

40. Haight, F., *Handbook of The Poisson Distribution* (New York 1967), 121.

41. McKendrick, A.G., 'Studies on the Theory of Continuous Probabilities, with special reference to its Bearing on Natural Phenomena of a Progressive Nature' in *Proc. Lond. Math. Soc.* (1914), *13*, 401-16.

42. Bartlett, M.S., *Stochastic Process* (Cambridge 1955), 54.

43. McKendrick, A.G., 'The rise and fall of epidemics' in *Paludism* (1912) *I*, 54-66.

44. Ross Archives, Letter dated 5 December 1912 from A.G. McKendrick to R. Ross.

45. *ibid.*

46. *The Indian Medical Gazette* (October 1919), 396.

47. Ritchie, J., *History of the Laboratory of the Royal College of Physicians of Edinburgh* (Edinburgh 1953).

48. McKendrick, A.G., 'Applications of mathematics to medical problems' in *Proc. Edin. Math. Soc.* (1926), *44*, 98-130.

49. Irwin, J.O., 'The place of mathematics in medical and biological studies' in *Jou. Roy. Statist. Soc.* (1963), *A,* 1–45.

50. Connolly, B.W. and Oliviera-Pinto, F., *Applicable Mathematics of Non-physical Phenomena* (New York 1982.)

51. Kermack, W.O. and McKendrick, A.G., 'Contributions to the mathematical theory of epidemics, I-V' in *Proc. Roy. Soc.* (1927), *A115*, 700-21; *Proc. Roy. Soc.* (1932), *A138*, 55-82; *Proc. Roy. Soc.* (1933), *A161*, 94-122; *Jou. Hygiene* (1937), *37*, 172-87; *Jou. Hyg.* (1939), *39*, 271-288.

52. Ritchie, *op.cit.*, 72-3.

53. Mollison, D., 'The importance of demographic stochasticity in population dynamics' in Hiorns, R.W. and Cooke, D.L., (eds.), *The Mathematical Theory of the Dynamics of Biological Populations* (London 1977), 97-107.

54. Kermack, W.O. and McKendrick, A.G., 'Some properties of points arranged at random on a Möbius surface' in *Mathematical Gazette* (1938), *22*, 66-72.

55. 'A Mathematical Curiosity. Properties of a "Möbius Surface"' in *The Scotsman* (6 March 1937).

56. Harvey, W.F., obituary notice (see note 21 above), 500-6.

57. McKendrick, A.G., 'House infection in cholera and cancer' in *Edin. Med. Jou.* (1923), *30*, 53-61.

58. *British Medical Journal* (30 December 1922), 1266.

59. Ross Archives, Letter dated 6 August 1911 from A.G. McKendrick to R. Ross.

60. Kendall, D.G., 'Stochastic processes and population growth' in *Jou. Roy. Statist. Soc.* (1949), *B11,* 230-82.

61. Bartlett, M.S., *op.cit.*

62. Irwin, J.O., *op.cit.*

63. Gani, J., 'The early use of stochastic methods: an historical note on McKendrick's pioneering papers' in Krishnaiah, P.R. (ed.), *Essays in Statistics and Probability* (North-Holland 1981), 1-5.

64. Hoppensteadt, F.C., 'Some influences of population biology on mathematics' in *Memoirs of the Amer. Math. Soc.* (1984), *48*, 25-9.

65. Tong, H., 'Art of the probable' in *South China Morning Post* (6 April 1984).

66. Ross Archives, Letter dated 20 December 1911 from R. Ross to A.G. McKendrick.

67. Ross Archives, Letter dated 5 December 1912 from A.G. McKendrick to R. Ross.

Scotland and Australasia

D A Dow

1. Richards, Eric, 'Australia and the Scottish Connection, 1788-1914' in Cage, R.A., (ed.), *The Scots Abroad. Labour, Capital, Enterprise, 1750-1914* (London 1985), 111.

2. Richards, Eric, 'Varieties of Scottish Emigration in the Nineteenth Century' in *Historical Studies* (1985), *21*, No. 85, 173-94.

3. In Cage, *op.cit.*, 134. Richards' findings are confirmed by those of D.S. Macmillan who calculated that 28 of the 532 applications to settle in New South Wales and Van Diemen's Land between 1814–30 came from medical men — the sixth largest occupational grouping. Not all of these men were intent on clinical careers. Macmillan also demonstrated that 22 of the 416 original partners in the 1840 Scottish Australian Company were physicians or surgeons. See Macmillan, D.S., *Scotland and Australia, 1788-1850* (Oxford 1967), 102, 345.

4. Kiernan, Colm, (ed.), *Australia and Ireland 1788-1988: Bicentenary Essays* (Dublin 1986).

5. MacDonagh, O., 'Emigration from Ireland to Australia: An Overview' in Kiernan, *op.cit.*, 129.

6. More than twenty years ago the opening sentence of Macmillan's study recorded that 'The early connexion between Scotland and Australia has received less attention from historians than it deserves'. Macmillan, *op.cit.*, Introduction. The same might still be said of the Scottish doctors.

7. *Glas. Med. Jou.* (1884) *II*, 120.

8. Cited in Hamilton, David, *The Healers. A History of Medicine in Scotland* (Edinburgh 1981), 148, 151, 295 n.2, 296 n.3.

9. Young, J.A., Sefton, A.J. and Webb, N., (eds.), *Centenary Book of the University of Sydney Faculty of Medicine* (Sydney 1984), 24.

10. The discrepancies in the totals are accounted for by the fact that 59 individuals held qualifications from two separate Scottish cities, and two had collected degrees or diplomas from 3 of the 4.

11. Skirving, R.S., 'Surgery and Surgeons in Edinburgh over Forty years Ago' in *Med. Jou. Aust.* (1926), *I*, 295.

12. *Glas. Med. Jou.* (1884), *I*, 220.

13. Addison, W. Innes, *A Roll of the Graduates of the University of Glasgow* (Glasgow 1898), *passim*.

14. Moscucci, Ornella, 'The Science of Woman: British Gynaecology 1849-1890' (Oxford DPhil 1984), 38.

15. Dyason, Diana, 'James Jamieson and the Ladies' in Attwood, Harold and Home, R.W. (eds.), *Patients Practitioners and Techniques* (Melbourne 1985), 15.

16. *ibid*. The manuscript matriculation albums are retained in Glasgow University Archives.

17. Russell, K.F., *The Melbourne Medical School 1862-1962* (Melbourne 1977), 108. It is instructive to note that Glasgow University appointed its inaugural Professor of Clinical Medicine, (Sir) Thomas McCall Anderson, only in 1874, nine years after Jamieson graduated. The lack of such a position had long been regarded as one of the weaknesses of the Glasgow Medical School.

18. Wright-St Clair, R.E., 'The Edinburgh influence on New Zealand medicine' in *Proceedings of the XXIII International Congress of the History of Medicine* (London 1974), *Vol. 2*, 750.

19. Jones, D.W.C., *Annals of the University of Otago Medical School 1875-1939* (Wellington 1945), 82.

20. Russell, *op.cit.*

21. Brooking, Tom, '"Tam McCanny and Kitty Clydeside" — The Scots in New Zealand' in Cage, *op.cit.*, 156.

22. In Cage, *op.cit.*, 111.

23. Howard, G.T., 'Port Phillip's Early Doctors, 1835-1839' in *Med. Jou. Aust.* (1934), *I*, 365.

24. *The Medical Directory* (1857), 167.

25. The fluctuating fortunes of this movement for the study of Australian medical history are detailed in Forster, Frank M.C., '30 Years On. Medical History Society, 1953-83' in Attwood, Harold, Forster, Frank and Gandevia, Bryan (eds.), *Occasional Papers on Medical History Australia* (Melbourne 1984), 157-99. Scots appear to have played a prominent part in these early efforts. In 1902 T.P. Anderson Stuart, inaugural Dean of the Faculty of Medicine at the University of Sydney, expressed a desire to see a course in medical history added to the medical curriculum. See *Australasian Med. Gaz.* (1921), *21*, 501. Almost a quarter of a century later R.S. Skirving, another Scotsman and Edinburgh graduate, became the first President of the newly-formed section of Medical History and Literature of the New South Wales Branch of the British Medical Association. See *Med. Jou. Aust.* (1925), *I*, 634.

26. Fisher, Richard B., *Joseph Lister 1827-1912* (London 1977), 62-3.

27. For details of Pringle's years in N.S.W. see Brown, K.M. *Medical Practice in Old Parramatta* (Sydney 1937), 76-99.

28. Clark, C.M.H., *A History of Australia, Volume IV, 1851-88* (Melbourne 1978), 239.

29. Brown, *op.cit.*, 83-5,

30. Lister was resident in Edinburgh (1853-60), Glasgow (1860-9) and

Edinburgh again (1869-77) before removing to London. Both Scottish cities have consistently laid claim to him as one of *their* most illustrious practitioners.

31. O'Sullivan, David M., 'William Gillbee (1825-1885) and the Introduction of Antiseptic Surgery to Australia' in *Med. Jou. Aust.* (1966), *II*, 871–8; 'The Introduction of Antiseptic Surgery to Australia' in *Med. Jou. Aust.* (1967), *II*, 896–902.

32. O'Sullivan, *op.cit., Med. Jou. Aust.* (1966), *II*, 875.

33. Malloch, a native of Canada, graduated MB (1867) and MD (1869), both Glasgow. He filled the coveted post of house surgeon to Lister in 1867–8. Malloch published a series of reminiscences of his old Chief on the latter's death in 1912. See *Lister Centenary Exhibition at the Wellcome Historical Medical Museum. Handbook* (London 1927), 171.

34. O'Sullivan, *op.cit., Med. Jou. Aust.* (1966), *II*, 876.

35. *ibid.*; O'Sullivan, *op.cit., Med. Jou. Aust.* (1967), *II*, 899.

36. *New South Wales Med. Gaz.* (1872), *II*, No. 12, 372.

37. Obituary notice of J.H. Pringle, *Glas. Med. Jou.* (1941), *I*, 153-7.

38. Duguid, Charles, *Macewen of Glasgow. A Recollection of the Chief* (Edinburgh 1957), 150-1.

39. Macewen's correspondence from Australia can be found in the Macewen Papers in Glasgow University Archives, DC79/16 and DC79/25.

40. Duguid, *op.cit.*

41. A detailed and very readable account of these early developments at the G.R.I. is Smith, Christopher, 'Medical radiology: its practical application 1895-1914' in Checkland, Olive and Lamb, Margaret (eds.), *Health Care as Social History: The Glasgow Case* (Aberdeen 1982), 100-16.

42. *Salute to the X-Ray Pioneers of Australia* (Sydney 1946), 19, 26. None of the articles was signed, other than the foreword by Sir Lawrence Bragg, Cavendish Professor of Physics, Cambridge.

43. *ibid.*, 34.

44. *ibid.*, 47. It is stated that this announcement appeared in the *British Medical Journal* of 20 June 1896. Despite a careful search, I have been unable to locate the quotation.

45. F.H. Quaife seems to have kept in touch with at least some of his Glasgow contemporaries, including Joseph Coats, Professor of Pathology in the University of Glasgow from 1893-9 and Pathologist to the Western Infirmary, where Donald Mackintosh held the post of Medical Superintendent. Coats visited the Antipodes in a vain attempt to restore his health in 1898, and recorded in great detail his reunions with Quaife and numerous other Glasgow graduates. See Coats, Joseph, *Notes on Sea and Land: A Diary* (Glasgow 1898), *passim.*

46. Young *et al.*, *op.cit..*, 73-5.

47. Interestingly, Kelvin had acted as one of the appointing committee when a Professor of Physics was elected to the University of Sydney in March 1886. The extent of his influence on Australian radiology might be revealed in the voluminous Kelvin correspondence which is deposited in Cambridge University Library (Ms.Add. 7342).

48. *Salute*, 49-51: *Australian Dictionary of Biography Volume 9: 1891-1939* (Melbourne 1983), 183-4. The London Hospital reference is puzzling, for the Hospital at that time had no medical electrician, unlike the G.R.I. and other leading UK institutions. See Clark-Kennedy, A.C., *The London, A Study in the Voluntary Hospital System* (London 1963), *Vol. 2*, 125.

49. Forster, *op.cit.*, 160.

50. Gandevia, Bryan, 'The Pattern of Australian Medical History' in *Proc. Roy. Soc. Med.* (1957), *50*, 591.

American Jewish Medical Students
in Scotland 1925–40
K E Collins

1.   'Review of the Year 5690' in *American Jewish Year Book* (1930-1), *32*,78-9.

2. *ibid.*

3. 'Review of the Year 5695' in *Amer. Jew. Y.B.* (1935-6), *37*, 157-8.

4. Silbermann, Charles, *A Certain People* (New York 1985), 53.

5. Synnot, Marcia Graham, *The Half Opened Door: Discrimination and Admissions at Harvard, Yale and Princeton 1900-1970* (Westport 1979), 14.

6. *ibid.,* 60.

7. Steinberg, Stephen, 'How Jewish Quotas Began' in *Commentary* (1971), *52*, 72.

8. Synnot, *op.cit.*, 160.

9. 'In the Matter of Race Discrimination at Rutgers University' — a complaint before the New Jersey State Board of Regents, 1930-1.

10. Flexner, Abraham, *Medical Education in the United States and Canada* (New York 1910).

11. Jarcho, Saul, 'Medical Education in the United States: 1910-1956' in *Journal of the Mount Sinai Hospital, Vol. XXXVI*, No. 4, 357-8.

12. 'Review of the Year 5691' in *Amer. Jew. Y.B.* (1931-2), *33,*55-6.

13. Rosenberg, Charles, (ed.), *Healing and History: Essays for George Rosen* (New York 1979), 250.

14. Pearle, Kathleen, *Preventive Medicine: the Refugee Physician and the New York Medical Community 1933-1945* (Bremen 1981), 32.

15. See the 'Annual Reports on Medical Education and Licensure' in *Jou. Amer. Med. Ass.* (1933-40).

16. *Jou. Amer. Med. Ass.* (1935), *104*, 1055.

17. Bloomgarden, Lawrence, *A Preliminary Analysis of Discrimination Against Jewish Applicants for Admission to Medical School in New York State* (published privately by American Jewish Committee 1952), 18-24.

18. Wechsler, Harold, *The Qualified Student* (New York 1977), 169.

19. Oren, Dan, *Joining the Club: A History of the Jews and Yale* (New York 1985), 149.

20. *Jou. Amer. Med. Ass.* (1935), *104*, 1054.

21. Personal communications with the author.

22. 'Medical Schools in Scotland' in *Brit. Med. Jou.* (1937), *II*, 476-8.

23. Weidman, Jerome, 'May 27, 1939 — Royal Bank of Scotland, St. Andrews Square, Edinburgh, Scotland — $50' in *Letter of Credit* (New York 1940), 111.

24. See Sir Hector Hetherington's reference to 'less desirable aliens' in Illingworth, Sir Charles, *University Statesman: Sir Hector Hetherington* (Glasgow 1971), 55.

25. Braverman, Harold, 'Medical School Quotas' in *Barriers: Patterns of Discrimination Against Jews* (New York n.d.), 74-7.

26. Minutes of the General Council for 1930: see Appendix XII (Interim Report of the Colonial and Foreign Students Committee, on the Applications of American students to study medicine in Great Britain and Ireland), 317-8; Memorandum of the Registrar, Norman C. King, on the American Medical Students, 319-23; Memorandum on Registration of Students (Norman Walker), 324-7; Reports of the Scottish Branch of the General Medical Council, 455-62.

27. Minutes of the G.M.C. (1932), 5.

28. Personal communication from Dr. Robert Smart, Keeper of the Muniments, University of St Andrews Library.

29. Personal communications with the author.

30. Personal communication from Phil Kozinn, President, St Andrews American Medical Alumni Association.

31. *Jou. Amer. Med. Ass.* (1939), *113*, 772.

32. *Lister Journal*, [the journal of the extra-mural medical colleges of medicine in Glasgow] (Glasgow 1940), *Vol. 2*, No. 2, 18.

33. *Jewish Echo* (issues of 15, 22, 29 November and 6 December 1935).

34. *ibid.* (20 April 1935).

35. Daiches, David, *Two Worlds: An Edinburgh Jewish Childhood* (Sussex 1971), 127-8.

36. Goldberg, Jacob A., 'Jews in Medicine' in *Medical Economics* (March 1940), 56.

37. *Comments of the Governing Board of the Medical School of the Royal Colleges of Edinburgh on the Report of The Goodenough Committee on the Future of Non-University Medical Schools* (Edinburgh, privately printed), 2.

38. Hamilton, David, *The Healers: A History of Medicine in Scotland* (Edinburgh 1981), 273.

Index